BIRD FLU
ARE YOU
PREPARED?

A Practical Guide to Homœopathic Treatment for Bird Flu

by

Henrietta Wells *MCH, RSHom.*

AF732730

Published by Henrietta Wells
Publishing partner: Paragon Publishing, Rothersthorpe
First published 2007

ISBN 1-899820-29-0

Book design, layout and production management by Into Print
www.intoprint.net
Printed and bound in UK and USA by Lightning Source

Disclaimer
The author assumes that all readers understand any risks involved with advice within this book and accepts no liability whatsoever.

With gratitude to Andrew Wells TD,
www.mere-house.co.uk, editorial consultant.

* * *

In memory of my sister Julia Luard 1.2.51-15.7.07 RIP.

* * *

Author biography

Henrietta Wells is a very experienced homœopath who has been practising for many years; since 1987 she has been based in Wiltshire where people come from all over the UK and abroad to see her. Most of her homœopathic knowledge was gained from the renowned homœopath the late Dr Margery Blackie C.V.O. in the 1970s as well as at the College of Homœopathy in London.

In 1993 her first book *Homœopathy for Children* was published and in 2002 her second book *Homœopathy: The Modern Prescriber*. This latter book covers the homœopathic treatment for acute diseases such as Whooping Cough, Chickenpox, Measles, Mumps etc., as well as instructions for treating many injuries such as bites, stings, sunstroke, burns, broken bones and wounds; it also gives advice about the treatment of coughs, colds, earaches, exam anticipation nerves, head lice, hangovers, malaria prevention, DVT risks when flying and much more.

Contents

SECTION ONE

Chapter One
Is there really a threat or is it simply scaremongering? 8
Homœopathic successes when treating acute diseases, epidemics and pandemics 10
Immunity and susceptibility 12
What would happen if there were a pandemic? 14

Chapter Two
How homœpathy began and what it is 16
Making homœopathic remedies – homœopathic potencies 19
Care of homœopathic remedies 20
Buying homœopathic remedies 21
Storage and travelling with homœopathic remedies 22

Chapter Three
Bird flu symptoms 24
Early stages of Bird flu 24
As Bird flu develops 25
Taking the homœopathic case 26
Heirarchy of symptoms 28
Repertorization 29

Chapter Four
Some demonstration cases 31
Comparison of some remedies 43
Patient record chart 45
Repertorization chart 46

Chapter Five
Prescribing the remedies and the size of the dose 47
Frequency of prescribing remedies 47
Signs of improvement 47
Signs of relapsing 48
Choosing the potency 48
Some other important rules on potencies and prescribing 49

Plussing a remedy 50
General nursing care when using homœopathy 51

Chapter Six
Homœopathic prevention of Bird flu 52
Making a nosode out of Bird flu 54
Prevention and treatment using Bird Flu Nosode 30 55
Additional remedies and advice for the acute treatment of Bird flu 55
Genus Epidemicus 56
Comparing Bird flu with SARS 56
Practical Preparations 57
Water purification, wound cleaning and general cleanliness 58

Chapter Seven
Remedies for any after-effects of Bird flu 59
Dosage for after Bird flu remedies 60
Relationships for after-effects remedies 61

SECTION TWO

Homœopathic Bird Flu Repertory 62

SECTION THREE

Homœopathic Materia Medica for Bird Flu 88
Aconite 88
Antim.Tart. 90
Apis 91
Argent. Nit. 91
Arsenicum Album 92
Arsenicum Iodatum 93
Baptisia 93
Belladonna 94
Bryonia 95
Camphora 96
Carbolic Acid 97
Carbo Veg. 97
Chelidonium 98
Crotalus Horridus 99
Eup. Perf. 100
Ferrum Phos. 100
Gelsemium 101

Hepar Sulph. 102
Ipecac. 103
Kali Carb. 103
Lachesis 104
Merc. Sol or Merc. Viv. 105
Muriatic Acid. 106
Natrum Sulph. 107
Nitric Acid 107
Nux Vomica 108
Oscillococcinum (Anas. Barb.) 109
Phosphorus 109
Pulsatilla 110
Pyrogen 111
Rhus Tox. 112
Sanguinaria 113
Sulphur 114
Veratrum Album 115
Veratrum Viride 115

Appendix
Remedy names 117

Section One

Chapter One

Is there really a threat or is it simply scaremongering?

In the 20th century there were three flu pandemics and each originated from birds. The first in 1918, Spanish flu, killed somewhere between 30 and 40 million people worldwide. In 1957 Asian flu killed two million people worldwide and in 1968 Hong Kong flu killed one million people worldwide. It is not surprising that with this history of other types of Bird flu, scientists are concerned about H5N1. The 1918 pandemic is thought to have been much worse because it occurred at the end of the First World War when millions of soldiers were returning home, thus spreading it far and wide in a way that did not happen in 1957 and 1968.

In order to decide whether there is a genuine threat or not, we need to look at the facts of this disease. So far it appears to have spread only from birds to people and has never yet mutated so that it is being spread from human to human. When it is only spread from domestic birds to humans it is relatively easy to control by culling birds, and also by keeping domestic birds indoors so that they do not infect the wild fowl population. There is relatively little to worry about from the pandemic point of view while this is still the case, even though Bird flu is serious and kills approximately 50% of those who catch it. However, as the wild fowl population is becoming more widely infected this is an added reason for concern because it is being spread over a much wider geographical area, but you would still need to have close contact with an infected bird to catch the disease. The risk is increased during times of migration when the wild fowl population spreads it to new areas. It has already spread from Southeast Asia to Western China, Mongolia, Kazakhstan, and Eastern and Western Europe.

Everyone who has caught Bird flu is thought to have had close contact with infected birds. The Bird flu virus is one against which humans are known to have no immunity at all, as we can see from the devastating effects on those who have caught it. It is only when someone already carrying a human-to-human flu virus catches Bird flu, that the two viruses could merge and this would result in a human-to-human strain of Bird flu. The moment this happens, that is when it mutates into a form which can infect via human-to-human contact (not just bird to human contact as at present), will be the time when it will become really worrying. This is because it can then be spread worldwide within a matter of days via air travel. Obviously air travel has increased dramatically since the pandemics of 1918, 1957 and 1968, and this would put many more people at risk much faster than previously; it is unlikely that there will be any time to contain it. As mentioned earlier, the reason the 1918 outbreak killed many more people than the other two pandemics was mainly due to the large numbers of soldiers returning home from fighting in the First World War. Today's air travel is the modern day equivalent of such large numbers of people on the move, only that travelling is much quicker now, with a consequently faster spread of the disease.

Since genes can mutate when Bird flu comes in contact with a human who already has ordinary flu, this is most likely to occur in someone having close contact with domestic birds. However, other sources of contact with it have been discovered. For instance it was found in some fertilizer made from chicken waste (from infected birds) in Indonesia. It has recently been reported that it is affecting a chicken farm in the UK, spread by importing semi-processed turkey which had been infected with the Bird flu virus. Another source is from pigs which are also capable of catching ordinary flu, usually known as Swine flu. Just as in a human, if a pig becomes infected with both viruses at the same time, the two viruses could mutate and produce a new virus easily passed from person to person. So there are now many possible sources where Bird flu can "join" with human flu and mutate into one that can be caught by human-to-human contact: those in contact with domestic birds, those in contact with contaminated fertilizer or infected imported semi-processed food, those in contact with contaminated wild fowl and those in contact with contaminated pigs. Any of these sources, could increase the risk of mutation from bird-to-human Bird flu to human-to-human Bird flu, which is most likely to result in a pandemic.

Millions of tiny viruses are spread through the air at every sneeze with ordinary flu. These land on many surfaces and can survive for as long as two days. Any contact, be it by touch or breathing in the virus, can result in flu. The difference with Bird flu, unlike ordinary flu, is that statistically so far it has been shown to kill approximately 50% of its victims, so not only does it spread at great speed but it is also much more destructive than other types of flu. There has been much research into the various flu viruses and they have now been able to collect tissue samples preserved from the 1918 outbreak; it has been discovered that the 1918 virus has some similar characteristics to the H5N1 virus. The disease in 1918 also had many symptoms similar to today's H5N1 virus such as the patient appearing blue or even black from lack of oxygen. This may occur when pneumonia develops and lung tissue breaks down. Another major symptom recorded from both 1918 Spanish flu and H5N1 is bleeding from any part of the body; eyes, nose, mouth, ears, lungs and skin, as well as vomiting blood, having bloody expectoration, and bloody stools and urine.

Influenza by its very nature appears to be constantly mutating, and as it takes several months to create a new vaccine, it is very difficult for scientists to develop any vaccine to deal with any current, or new, strain. At present they have to develop a new vaccine annually, and quite often even this is inadequate because they cannot keep pace with the speed at which the virus mutates. An added problem is that vaccines lose potency if they spend too long sitting on the shelf unused. Routine testing uncovered the fact that this has already begun to happen with some of the earliest experimental vaccines against Bird flu.

It would be naive to assume that the hospitals and medics in this country could cope with a Bird flu pandemic. While they are hard working and very willing, the sad fact is that they have virtually no treatments known to be successful, and could only provide nursing care, respirators and so on. Such treatment would be very limited because there simply are not enough beds, nor is there enough equipment, to deal with the kind of demand that would be likely during a pandemic. No one knows whether or not Tamiflu or Relenza, the allopathic (conventional) treatments for flu, will work against human-to-human Bird flu, as they have never been able to be tested against Bird flu. It is thought that even if they prevent actual death, **they will *not* prevent extremely serious illness, and may well *cause* very serious long-term side-effects and after-effects.** There have been many reports of adverse reactions to Tamiflu, which include hallucinations, self-injury, abnormal and strange behaviour or what is known as "psychiatric adverse events". It has apparently killed over 150 people so far (to 2006). Some initial reactions can include respiratory failure, jaundice, nausea, vomiting, inflammation of the pericardium which causes chest pain and an abnormally rapid heart beat, and ultimately, occasionally, death. Roche Canada says Tamiflu has a good "safety profile" and emphasize that no causal relationship between any abnormal behaviour or adverse reactions have been linked to the drug. *However, all these side-effects and other information is readily available on the internet.* It is unimaginable that anyone would really want to take a drug once they know that even its minor side-effects while taking it are horrible, its efficacy against Bird flu unproven and questionable, and the after-effects of the treatment known to be long lasting and damaging to the system; all this is bad enough, quite apart from the fact that it can also occasionally cause death.

This is one of the reasons this book has been written, as with correctly chosen homœopathic remedies none of these problems should become an issue, because all the symptoms should be able to be cured with carefully chosen homœopathic remedies.

Homœopathic successes when treating acute diseases, epidemics and pandemics

One of the advantages about homœopathic treatment is that it is not essential to have a diagnosis in order to treat someone. This is because while it is the *common* symptoms (the ones that typically most people have) that lead to the diagnosis of a disease which is required for conventional medical treatment, it is the symptoms that *differentiate* one person's suffering with the disease from the next, which lead to the choice of homœopathic treatment. You could, for instance, have twenty people with mumps and they could all end up with different remedies because their individual symptoms are different from each other. In one person the glandular swelling could start on the left, in another person it could start on the right, another person could have incredibly smelly breath, while another might find that it mostly affects the testes. Another person could have severe mastitis with red streaks radiating from the centre, another could be desperately thirsty with very dry lips, while someone else could be thirstless and craving for fresh air. Yet another person could have pains shooting into the ear, or mastitis that is stony hard with pains spreading all over the body. So you treat the **individual's unique group of symptoms** which will differ from person to person, rather than the actual disease diagnosis (which is the name given to the common symptoms of a disease). Any of these descriptions could fit people who have mumps, but they are all different, and would need different remedies. *If you prescribe the similar remedy to the symptoms, that is, the remedy that is homœopathic to that particular individual, you should have success; it does not matter what the diagnosis is particularly, because that is the least important symptom of them all. This is the reason why you can prescribe homœopathically for Bird flu, or any other condition for that matter, even if you have never come across it before and do not know what it is. It is helpful, of course, to have a proper diagnosis, as one then knows how a disease may progress and change, but it is the least important piece of information required when treating someone homœopathically. This book enables you to choose the homœopathic remedy that fits the symptom picture presented by any individual with severe flu or pneumonia, and any other symptoms which could indicate Bird flu.*

In 1854 there was a cholera outbreak in London. The death rate was 54% in conventional hospitals but 16% in the London Homœopathic Hospital. (Ref. Dr. Dorothy Shepherd.) The mortality rate of cholera was about 50 to 60% in those days, yet during epidemics in New York and Europe, in patients having homœopathic treatment, the death rate was around 9%. In 1830-31 statistics on cholera treatment in Russia published by the Foreign Ministry showed a 63% mortality rate from allopathic treatment and an 11% mortality rate from homoeopathic treatment. (Ref. Alexander Ostrovsky, Ollo Homeopathic Center, Korolev-10, Moscow Region, 141070 Russia.) In 1836 in Vienna, it appeared that while two-thirds of the cases treated homœopathically by Dr. Fleischmann recovered, two-thirds of those treated by the ordinary methods in the other hospitals died. (Ref. Sir William Wilde in his work on Austria.) In the *Homœopathic World* of July 1889, it gives the comparative statistics of the treatment of the epidemic which affected Melbourne, Australia, in the first three months of that year. The following is a list of the cases treated at three hospitals, two of them allopathic (conventional) with the number of deaths and percentage in each case. They are taken from the *Melbourne Herald* of April 29th, 1889:-

	No of Beds	Typhoid cases	Deaths	%
Melbourne Hospital	318	431	78	18.1
Alfred Hospital	144	324	50	15.4
Homœopathic Hospital	60	305	22	7.1

In the records of three years of diphtheria in Broome County, NY from 1862 to 1864, there was a report of an 83.6% mortality rate among the allopaths and a 16.4% mortality rate among the homœopaths. (Ref. National Center for Homœopathy, 801 N. Fairfax Street, Suite 306 Alexandria, Virginia 22314.) During a meningococcus outbreak in Brazil in 1974, 18,640 patients were given the homœopathic nosode Meningococcinum as prophylaxis (preventative medicine) while 6,430 received no treatment. The treatment group reported 4 cases to 32 cases in the no treatment group (23 times more effective than no treatment). (Ref. National Center for Homœopathy.)

While the above are a minute sample of statistics from the past concerning homœopathic treatment and its successes, there are a vast number of current statistics. These and a great deal of information can be found on the internet on websites www.whale.to, www.homstudy.net, www.homeopathic.org, www.homeopathyresource.com, www.vaccinetruth.org, www.minimum.com, www.hpathy.com, www.homeopathy4everyone, and many others. The information should be very useful for those doubters of homœopathy. Those of us who are familiar with it, and have been practising it for years, have a wealth of knowledge and experience of its exciting and extraordinary successes.

Immunity and susceptibility

It is important to remember the relevance of one's susceptibility to succumbing to a disease. If our immune systems are healthy and have not been put into a constant state of alertness to fight disease through mass vaccination (which actually weakens the immune system) our bodies will be able to resist and be less susceptible to damage from viruses and bacteria. We should not be so concerned about the virus or the bacteria, but whether the soil (our bodies) in which the virus or bacteria finds itself is strong enough to resist. You could again pick twenty people with mumps: some will have it very badly, some mildly and some have symptoms somewhere in between these two. They will all have come into contact with the same bug, but they are reacting differently depending on their individual underlying health and susceptibility. Homœopathic treatment does not actually fight the virus or bacteria but helps the immune system throw off the disease, by choosing remedies which fit the individual's unique symptom picture. With Bird flu these individual symptoms will lead us to the choice of homœopathic remedy even if we have never seen the disease before. There should not really have to be any fear of the virus, but instead, one should have an observant attitude to enable one to choose the similar remedy. If the soil is healthy you should be able to throw the disease off with individualized help provided by the homœopathic remedies.

Many alternative health professionals and some homœopaths say that because the Western world is so highly vaccinated they will not "over-react" to Bird flu, nor will they get it very badly and produce the symptoms of the body destroying itself; that it is in the East, where there has been generally rather less vaccination that there will be this over-reaction and the more serious cases. This they suggest is because people are generally much healthier in the East because their immune systems have not had so much vaccination damage, and consequently their bodies would be robust enough to have a strong reaction. While it is certainly true that having less vaccination will make their immune systems stronger, I do not necessarily agree that that is the reason why young adults catch Bird flu more often, or the reason they get it more seriously, producing the more dangerous symptoms of the body attacking itself. First, we do not yet know whether or not it will only be the healthy young adults with strong immune systems who will over-react in this way. Second, the statistics show that currently healthy young adults are the age group most likely to be in contact with Bird flu as they are the ones most likely to be looking after birds. It does not necessarily mean they are more susceptible; it may simply mean they have closer and more frequent contact. During the pandemic of 1918 the age group which caught flu most then were the soldiers returning from war, and by doing so spread it far and wide. They were so-called fit young men. They were probably rather less fit at that time than those who had stayed at home; in fact most of them would have been thoroughly exhausted and run down. They were however, in contact with many, many more people, and a more varied selection of people, than those left at home, so consequently had far more opportunity to come into contact with flu. In addition they had frequently been living or travelling in large groups in confined spaces, where the spread would have been extremely fast. In other words, both in the flu epidemic of 1918, and now with Bird flu caught from birds the so-called healthy young adults who caught it most, and are catching it most, were and are the ones who have had much more opportunity, closer and more frequent contact. Also, it follows that the age group most frequently affected will have correspondingly higher numbers of serious cases, when the body starts destroying itself. I think what actually is going on is that when the very destructive miasm, (inherited weakness, or disposition) is currently most active in any individual it causes them to over-react and the body to self destruct, rather than being due to them being super healthy. It should be possible to prevent the body destroying itself by using homœopathic remedies, and this is described in Chapter Six on prevention.

One other point is that in the heavily vaccinated population in the West today, there can still be a strong response, or "over-reaction", to a "germ", despite the greatly increased vaccination programmes. This can happen in scarlet fever and in chicken pox, as well as with some of the other childhood diseases, despite the individuals having been vaccinated.

What would happen if there were a pandemic?

No one knows whether or not Tamiflu or Relenza will work against human-to-human Bird flu as they have never been able to be tested. It is thought that even if they prevent actual death, they will not prevent extremely serious illness and very serious long-term, possibly new, after-effects in those who get Bird flu badly. It is already known that Bird flu affects some people very seriously, causing death, while others get it relatively mildly; and although some may be very ill during the acute disease, they can recover well. There is no reason to suppose that human-to-human Bird flu will be very different in its effects. With homœopathic treatment there should be no long-term serious after-effects since the homœopathic remedies stimulate the patient to fight the disease, rather than impose a drug layer on top of an already serious illness, as happens with conventional treatment. The problem with emergency vaccines, if there are any spare and suitable for the disease, which is unlikely, is that of long-term side-effects too numerous to mention. This would be even more of a problem if they are untried and untested, and side-effects in large numbers have occurred whenever there has been mass immunization. For instance, in 1976 the disease known as Guillain-Barre Syndrome affected many of those vaccinated. This is polyneuritis with progressive muscular weakness of the limbs that can lead to paralysis. Probably only the medics would be given any vaccinations anyway, and it is questionable if that is a good idea. Also it takes up to about six months to produce enough of a vaccine after a new strain of flu has emerged. This involves using a large supply of chicken eggs, which will no doubt be unavailable as not only do they have to be ordered in advance, but most chickens will probably be dead due to Bird flu; both from the disease itself but also from culling.

However, it is important to plan ahead to minimize the problems which may occur. If you look at the aftermath of serious hurricanes or earthquakes, those suffering in the area are almost totally dependant on outside help. Many die while they are waiting to be rescued, fed, watered and protected from the elements, as well as from any injuries or diseases which may have resulted from the trauma. With a flu pandemic the hospitals could be overflowing with patients within a few days. The sick would be being looked after by thoroughly exhausted medics due to a shortage of staff and from working long hours; people no doubt will be told to stay at home as much as possible. Since the spread of the disease is fast, and the speed with which serious symptoms may develop is also very fast, there could be such huge numbers of people suddenly suffering from very serious life threatening symptoms, that there could be no time to get any professional assistance. Even if there were time to seek some kind of treatment, with hospitals full to bursting point there may be no help available; travel could be impossible or even prohibited in a futile last ditch attempt to prevent a pandemic. This situation could continue for many months. In the worst scenario, public transport, supplies of petrol and food, post deliveries, rubbish collections and many other services, which we expect as a matter of course, may stop for a while. It may sound ridiculous and alarmist, but you could well need to have a supply of food which will last you a minimum of three months, although it is probably best to be prepared for it to last much longer. This is not only so that you do not have to go out and run the risk of contact with Bird flu, but more importantly because there may well not be any, or only a few, supplies in the shops. People tend to think there will always be someone around to turn to, or to rescue them, in a dire situation, but with Bird flu there will probably be very little, if any, help available. **Your survival might well be down to you and you alone.**

Chapter Two

How Homœopathy began and what it is

The most common thing people think they know about homœopathy is that the dose of the substances used to make each remedy is so minute and tiny that it is totally useless; that for this reason it is a ridiculous system and not worth considering for any type of illness, let alone for anything serious. When homœopathy was first introduced opinion was very different. The man behind it all, Samuel Hahnemann, was a doctor in Germany who was born in 1755. He was not very enthusiastic about the various medical treatments available at that time, in fact he was fairly horrified at some of the methods used as they seemed to make very little sense and most of them did not work; quite a number of them actually made the patient worse and on many occasions caused their death. For this reason he actually stopped practising as a doctor, and since he was also a brilliant linguist he earned his living translating medical texts, rather than continuing with the questionable medical methods of his day.

While doing all these translations he noticed that the very few medicines that did genuinely work at that time seemed to be made from substances that **actually caused similar symptoms to the ones they were supposed to be treating.** The fact that a substance that can cause particular symptoms in a healthy person could actually cure those same symptoms when met with in a sick person, was not a new idea. There had been much debate in Hahnemann's time and also since the days of Hippocrates, as to whether a substance producing similar effects, or a substance producing opposite effects, to the symptoms of a disease, would be most beneficial and curative. This fact is nearly always left out of the current debate about what homœopathic prescribing really involves and as to whether or not homœopathy works; all that conventional doctors and scientists concentrate on is the minuteness of the homœopathic dose, which they hold up to ridicule. It is almost as if they are afraid of looking at the real facts, that choosing a substance which can cause certain symptoms in a healthy person can also cure those same symptoms in a sick person. This is what homœopathy is all about and it is vital to understand this. Conventional medicine is by and large based on treating people using drugs producing opposing effects to the disease. An allopathic drug can be used to treat symptoms in a patient similar to its side-effects, which more or less amounts to using the drug homœopathically instead of allopathically; drugs can be found to be very effective when used in this way, although it is a somewhat rare event.

When substances are chosen for their similar effects to the symptoms presented by the patient, that is homœopathically, there is a problem with the likelihood of them causing an aggravation of the symptoms before the patient can improve, and obviously this could be highly dangerous. Hahnemann was rather stumped as to what to do about this since he knew that simply diluting the remedy would make it weaker and less effective, although he was having to do it this way at that time because he knew of no other method of prescribing the similar remedies. It was only by mistake that he came across the idea of diluting and successing a remedy. This happened by chance as some of his remedies fell out of his case when he was travelling and were rolling around on the carriage floor. When he next used these particular remedies on patients, he discovered that they were much more effective than the straightforward dilutions that he had been using previously. He was fascinated as to why this should be the case and being a methodical man he then decided to shake very vigorously each of his remedies at every stage of dilution. Succussion is the name given for shaking the bottle of the remedy very vigorously a particular number of times at each stage of dilution. This was his way of carrying out, as scientifically as possible, the equivalent of the remedy rolling around on the carriage floor. He found that the remedies not only continued to work, but worked even better when succussed, much more so than when they were simply just diluted. He proceeded to test all the remedies out in many different levels of dilution and succussion. As a result of all this testing of dilution **and** succussion he concluded that the more frequently a remedy is succussed the better it seems to work. This enabled the remedies to be made out of smaller and smaller quantities of material, which meant they were becoming safer and safer, while at the same time being succussed more and more so that they worked much more efficiently than previously.

It is very odd that many allopathic (conventional) doctors and scientists hold up to ridicule the minuteness of the dose while being at the same time terrified of the dangers of bacteria and viruses which are also minute. Quantum physics demonstrates that matter is not solid and inert as was originally thought and since the 1930s and 1940s experiments have shown that "during the accelerated collision process of particles, material particles are created and destroyed and their mass is transformed into energy". (See *Homœopathy: The Modern Prescriber* by Henrietta Wells ISBN 1-84293-027-3.) Quantum physics provides a possible explanation as to why a straightforward dilution of a substance simply makes the substance weaker, but dilution **with succussion** at every stage of the dilution appears to release some energy into the liquid remedy.

Yet another point to make to those who ridicule homœopathy because of the minuteness of the dose, is that it works very efficiently both on babies and animals. No baby or animal ever has any idea as to what remedy or drug it may be being given, yet with the appropriate remedy they still get better. There can be no explanation for this except for the fact that the similar (homœopathic) remedy **does** work and therefore the minuteness of the dose should not be considered a problem. You cannot call it a placebo reaction either, as that is also irrelevant when treating both babies and animals.

A remedy should always work if it is similar, that is homœopathic, to the symptoms presented by the patient. The difficulty lies in finding the most similar remedy. It can be a problem choosing a similar remedy if someone is not particularly ill and the symptoms are wishy washy and unclear, in which case it is probably best to wait and see what symptoms emerge which are unique to that person. It is also difficult if people are unable to describe in any detail the type of pain, emotions or other modalities that affect them. If someone refuses to tell you, or is very unhelpful, it is like them going to see an osteopath and leaving a few vertebrae at home; the osteopath would not be able to help. In the same way if someone is very vague or occasionally deliberately unhelpful in describing the symptoms, then it is almost impossible to choose the homœopathic remedy. In complicated cases where someone has many conditions or has had much suppression with conventional medicine it is also difficult to prescribe, but with patience and perseverance one can usually unravel the various layers of disease and the patient emerges a much healthier, happier person. As far as Bird flu is concerned the symptoms are dramatic and clear. There should not be too much of a problem choosing the homœopathic remedies required for cure.

When Hahnemann discovered the fact that like really does cure like, and also discovered that he could make all his remedies safe (regardless of how poisonous they may be in their original undiluted state) with the process of dilution and succussion, he set about experimenting with many different substances. This he did by getting groups of his friends to take small doses of a substance and noting down what symptoms they produced. The symptoms which they all produced from taking a particular substance were called provings of the remedies, and they were put together to form the basis for Hahnemann's Materia Medica. A Materia Medica is a summary of the symptoms each remedy can produce in healthy people. It consists of detailed pictures of symptoms of many remedies which, when met with in a sick person, will be truly curative. In Section Three of this book there are many remedy pictures, that is a Materia Medica, of the most likely remedies that could be curative in Bird flu.

In homœopathic prescribing the idea is to write down a detailed symptom picture of the patient, then re-write that list in order of importance, seriousness and severity. You fill out a Repertorization Chart (*see* Chapter Four) in order to discover which remedy or remedies are most similar to the suffering of the patient at that time. You then read up in more detail the remedies most indicated on the Repertorization Chart in the Materia Medica. This enables you to choose the most similar remedy, the homœopathic remedy, which should result in a cure. This is what this book sets out to do, to teach you how to do this and to look after yourself and your family at a time when there is no other known treatment which can be successful, and at a time when it is unlikely that anyone else will be able to help you.

Many people have used homœopathy before and will hopefully feel reasonably confident doing this. However, many others will be interested and keen, but not know where to start. This book will give you step-by-step instructions, but it would also be a good idea to get used to using homœopathic remedies and learn how to choose them for simple problems, perhaps First Aid type conditions, in order to learn the ropes. I suggest you read *Homœopathy: The Modern Prescriber* by Henrietta Wells (ISBN 1-84293-027-3) because it shows in a clear and straightforward way how you can treat things like burns, bites and stings, coughs, sore throats, fevers, and prevention and treatment of the childhood diseases. By doing this first you will become familiar with using homœopathy before Bird flu arrives. It would be sensible to find a local homœopath who could give you some homœopathic constitutional treatment to make sure you are as healthy as possible, and therefore more able to cope, when the time comes.

Making homœopathic remedies – homœopathic potencies

Homœopathic remedies are made starting with the mother tincture which is represented by this sign: Ø and is the undiluted original substance preserved in alcohol. The first dilution is made up of one drop of Ø and nine drops of alcohol which is successed or shaken to make the 1x. Nine drops of alcohol are mixed with one drop of the 1x and successed, to make the 2x. Nine drops of alcohol are mixed with one drop of the 2x and successed, to make the 3x. Nine drops of alcohol are mixed with one drop of the 3x and successed, to make the 4x, nine drops of alcohol are mixed with one drop of the 4x and successed to make the 5x and so on usually up to a 30x. These are the X range of potencies, that is, made up in dilutions of tenths. The X is always written after the number and can be in upper or lower case. The next range of potencies are the hundredths. Here the first dilution is made up of one drop of the Ø with 99 drops of alcohol and successed. This is 1C. 99 drops of alcohol are mixed with one drop of the 1C and successed, to make the 2C. 99 drops of alcohol are mixed with one drop of the 2C and successed to make the 3C. 99 drops of alcohol are mixed with one drop of the 3C and successed to make the 4C and so on until you get to the potency you want. Luckily all this is done by the pharmacist and you never have to do any of it but it is helpful to understand how they are made. With the hundredths range of potencies, the C range, the C can also be in upper or lower case, but in the C potencies the letter C after the potency number is often not written. This means that if someone refers to a remedy in a 30 that will **always** mean a 30C. It would never mean a 30x or 30M. The M range of potencies are obviously made in the same way and are thousandths, with succussion carried out at each step of the potentization. An M, usually written in upper case, will always follow the potency number to describe this range of potencies. Elsewhere in Europe they often use a D instead of an X, and cH or CH instead of C.

Some people get into a terrible muddle trying to understand the potency structure. They think a high potency number, that is a remedy in a high C or in the M range is stronger, or better, or more effective, than a lower potency. This is not actually the case. The higher the potency, the more energy it has, and therefore is more suited to a patient being very energetically sick, someone very cross, or restless or with a raging fever or screaming and so on, rather than someone who is sitting in a heap, scarcely moving, with no energy to talk much. It could follow that in general a child will have more energy and be more energetic, even when ill, than an elderly person might be when ill, so when treating a child one would be more likely to go for a higher potency, or expect to move up to a higher potency than for someone old. Obviously this is not always the case, there are plenty of energetic older people and lethargic younger people, but it is important to understand that **no one potency is better or stronger** or will work quicker than another; you **choose the potency to fit the energy of the patient,** meaning it must also be similar, or homœopathic, to the energy level of the patient. I will go into this in more detail when explaining treatment, but you need to grasp this idea first.

Care of homœopathic remedies

One of the rather tiresome things about having homœopathic treatment is that many things can antidote the remedies, but as they work so well, this minor problem is easily overcome and one gets used to it so that it becomes second nature. Since the dose is so tiny (and therefore wonderfully safe and without side-effects) you have to be careful how you store, handle and administer the remedies.

(1) Any strong taste or smell can antidote them. This means not taking the remedy close to any meal or drink as any strong taste will spoil them. Since the remedies work in the saliva, you suck them slowly and you should never wash them down with anything. The remedies taste of sugar, so are not at all unpleasant which is quite an advantage. Generally speaking you should allow a minimum of **20 minutes from your last meal**, but if it is urgent to take the remedy in an acute situation, like the ones to be described in this book, you should just go for it. It is highly unlikely, in an urgent situation with someone seriously ill, that they will have just eaten a strong tasting meal. Very bland food or drink, such as plain bread or water will have no detrimental effect on the remedy; for instance when prescribing for cattle, remedies are often put in their water, as their diet is relatively bland. The occasions when you should be very careful to allow the 20 minutes interval between eating or drinking and taking the remedy, are when you are having any long-term treatment from your homœopath. Therefore, while you should always try and stick to the 20 minute rule, in an acute situation take the remedy regardless as every second may count; just make sure **they are never washed down with a drink by a thirsty patient and are always taken in a clean mouth that has no taste in it, of food, drink or toothpaste.** In Chapter Seven, which covers the recovery afterwards, you should be careful to follow the 20 minute rule meticulously as you are then into the area of longer term treatment; there will no longer be any urgency so you can perfectly well wait 20 minutes or so.

(2) You should tip the remedy into the cap of the remedy bottle and from there chuck it into your mouth (rather than handling it) before sucking it slowly. You should be careful not to put the remedy cap close to the mouth as this can transfer infection as well as possibly antidote the remedies. I have noticed in my practice patients being very careless about this.

(3) You should never open the remedy bottle in a room where there is any strong smell, so do not open it in the kitchen if you have been peeling onions or in the bathroom if you have been using some strong smelling bath oil or salts. If you make a mistake about this, all the pills in the bottle could be antidoted; they could well not work, no longer be able to save lives, cure, or be relied upon in any way.

(4) Mobile telephones, cordless telephones as well as wi-fi computers can antidote remedies when switched on or used. *They need to be kept at least a metre away from the remedy* and you should never leave them close together.

(5) If you drop a remedy do not put it back into the bottle, throw it away as otherwise it could contaminate the rest of the pills in the bottle.

(6) Never transfer remedies from one bottle to another; always keep them in the original bottle. If you need to keep some separately for some reason, put them carefully in a clean envelope; then, when you need a dose, you should use a teaspoon to remove one from the envelope to put into the mouth.

(7) Substances to be avoided completely, as they very easily antidote homœopathic remedies, are coffee (decaffeinated is all right although it is not actually particularly good for you), peppermint, menthol, eucalyptus, camphor, Olbas Oil, tea tree oil and frankincense oil. Also generally be careful with all aromatherapy oils. Remember that many of these substances can be hidden in other things, such as in cough sweets, toothpastes, chest-rubs, teas and Vick. Camphor is often found in the heat rubs and ointments people use for muscular aches and pains and it will always antidote remedies.

Buying homœopathic remedies

Many remedies can be found now in health food shops and pharmacists, but for a condition such as Bird flu, when you might want remedies which you cannot find in such places, or may not be able to find them in the correct potency, it is best to have a supply kept in a sensible place in your home where they will not be spoiled. The following pharmacies send remedies through the post and are excellent.

Helios Homœopathic Pharmacy,
89-97 Camden Road, Tunbridge Wells, Kent. TN1 2QR.
Tel: 01892-536393
Email: pharmacy@helios.co.uk
Website: www.helios.co.uk

Ainsworths Homœopathic Pharmacy,
36 New Cavendish Street, London, W1G 8UF.
Tel: 0207 835 5330
Website: www.ainsworths.com

Galen Homeopathics,
Llewell Mill, West Stafford,
Dorchester, Dorset. DT2 8AN.
Tel: 01305 263996

Most of them will send up to about five remedies immediately, larger orders take a bit longer. You can get remedies in the form of soft pills which dissolve in the mouth immediately which are excellent for babies, but you do not get very many per bottle. They can also be in the form of hard flat tablets, or else in round balls, which are called pilules. Pilules are the best value for money but some people prefer the tablets. They all taste of sugar so there is no problem getting people to take them. You can also get them in liquid potencies which contain a small amount of alcohol.

Storage and travelling with homœopathic remedies

It is best to keep the remedies in a bedroom, well away from kitchen and bathroom smells, but also in a place where no one will tinker with them without you knowing, or inadvertently spoil them in some way and antidote them. As you may need to find a remedy in a hurry, have them standing upright with a label on the lid of each bottle (which is more legible than having them lying flat) and keep them in alphabetical order in some kind of box or tin; it is a good idea to make a cardboard grid to fit the box so that the bottles will not fall over. If you are worried about people going near them with a mobile telephone then you should keep them in a box kept in a lead lined bag to protect them from any damage from mobiles. Also if you happen to keep some with you in your pocket or bag then you should keep them in a lead lined bag because you never know when someone might pass near you with their mobile switched on. Lead lined bags can usually be obtained from camera shops as people use them to store their films. You can also get lead bags and lead fabric over the internet.

You should never let your remedies be x-rayed when going through security checks like those at airports. You can get a travel card from Helios Pharmacy which explains in many different languages that x-rays damage the remedies and that they should not go through them. While you may find some security people at airports who think they know best and will tell you that x-rays do not damage remedies, the fact remains that they are not homœopaths, they will be totally unaware that homœopathy can be used to treat and cure many serious conditions, so consequently may well think that it does not matter how the remedies are treated. They will often tell you that the radiation in the sky is just as damaging as the x-ray machine. There are statistics showing higher rates of cancer caused by radiation damage for radiologists because however careful they are they do get exposed to x-ray damage, but there has been no statistic showing this to be the case with frequent flyers or pilots, despite careful studies. This proves what we already know which is the fact that, *in the sky, the radiation wave length from the sun, is a totally different and less damaging frequency than those from x-ray machines.* The best thing to do when travelling is to keep the remedies in their box in the lead lined bag in your hand luggage, and when you are about to go through the metal detector security archway, hand the box of remedies to a security official with the travel card saying that they must not go through the x-ray. If you leave them in the lead lined bag to go through the x-ray machine those watching the screens will simply turn up the dial until it is strong enough to see through the lead lined bag, thus damaging the remedies which is what you most want to avoid.

Homœopathic remedies will last forever if looked after correctly so that they remain undamaged, although now, due to some European edict, there has to be a 'use by' date on them, which you can ignore, provided you care for the remedies properly. They are very good value, assuming they are not spoiled. Bearing in mind that the remedies really can and often do save lives (quite apart from preventing minor irritating conditions), it is extremely important to care for them sensibly; it should become automatic so that you can always rely on them.

Chapter Three

Bird flu symptoms

When Bird flu starts passing from person to person it will mean that the Bird flu virus had merged with the human flu virus, and that the infection could be carried far and wide very rapidly. It will mean that the infection initially only caught directly from birds will have mutated sufficiently to cause infection from person to person. This happens when a person who already has the human flu virus also catches Bird flu from contact with contaminated birds; Bird flu then mutates so that it would spread from that person to other people.

We do have quite a bit of detail about what happens when Bird flu is caught directly from birds themselves and it is reasonable to assume that Bird flu, once it has mutated and starts spreading from person to person, will have very strong similarities to those symptoms when it is caught from birds. The H5N1 type Bird flu virus has so far only jumped between species to infect people who have had close contact with infected birds. The flu virus is in birds' faeces, saliva and mucus and other birds catch it by contact with any of these, or inhaling the virus. Similarly people can inhale dried faeces which have been trampled into dust or when it sticks to feathers or other body parts of infected birds. Very close contact, usually with chickens but obviously with other birds, such as domestic ducks, is what puts humans at risk. As people would have acquired no natural immunity to the Bird flu virus, it could be very damaging and might cause many millions of deaths. Some people mistakenly think you can catch it from eating cooked birds, but this is not the case if they are cooked thoroughly at 165°C or higher.

The incubation period is thought to range from anything from two to eight days and apparently could be as long as 16 or 17 days. This is a bit longer than ordinary flu but once incubated the progression of the disease is very rapid.

Early stages of Bird flu

At the beginning, nearly everyone will have a fever, and/or chill, runny nose, headache and sore throat, just like any other kind of flu. The significant additional early features of Bird flu may include running a very high temperature (above 38°C), bleeding from the nose and/or gums, hoarse voice and perhaps conjunctivitis. It is impossible to say whether or not conjunctivitis arises simply because so far the people who have caught it from birds have lived at very close quarters with the dusty conditions of the domestic birds' habitat. It would be likely that such close contact could make them more likely to get eye infections. I have included these symptoms in the Materia Medica and the Repertory Sections of this book, as it may still be part of the overall Bird flu symptom picture when it has mutated into a human-to-human Bird flu. Certainly the eye symptoms are reported to become worse if the sufferer touches the eyes when they have Bird flu, which is an additional reason for frequent washing of the hands during an epidemic or pandemic.

As Bird flu develops

While Bird flu will begin as described above it may well develop in different ways affecting different bodily systems varying from individual to individual; there are four main areas that appear to be affected and the onset could take anything from a few hours to four or five days:-

(1) It may consist of chiefly intense, severe back and limb aches and pains of various types; or these may accompany symptoms described in (2) (3) or (4) below.

(2) There could be digestive problems with abdominal pain, nausea, vomiting and diarrhœa; typically the diarrhœa is very watery without much blood, but if the internal organs start breaking down, that is when the diarrhœa is likely to become much more bloody. Obviously the more diarrhœa there is, the more loss of fluid there is and the more dangerous the condition becomes.

(3) It could go down to the lungs developing into breathing problems, a crackling noise when breathing in, a cough and chest pains, and this may turn into pneumonia. Blood poisoning and destruction of lung tissue could follow, the lungs could fill up with fluid and breathing become difficult (and eventually impossible). When people cannot breathe properly they become what is known as cyanosed, which often shows as a purple, blue, grey, or even leaden skin colour, sometimes even described as black. This happens in Bird flu because of the lack of oxygen due to the breaking down of the lungs.

(4) Acute encephalitis (inflammation of the brain) often with delirium, particularly at the height of the fever, could occur, which may accompany some of the other symptoms described.

There is likely to be very extreme weakness and lethargy regardless which group of symptoms a person may have. Some people may have only one of these groups of symptoms but others could have some or all of them, in varying degrees of severity, at different stages of the infection, progressing from one to another; in Bird flu the progression is usually very fast. Sometimes these phases will merge and overlap so you should be very observant and aware of all the possibilities should the symptoms move on and change. When the body starts breaking down, that is when there could be multi-organ dysfunction, and there could be bleeding from anywhere; the mouth, eyes, nose, ears, anus, lungs and skin. This can apparently come on very quickly, sometimes within a day or even less, and death occurs very soon unless it is treated.

All these are the common symptoms of Bird flu. While there could be many people who have Bird flu who will be lucky enough to escape with just a very nasty dose of flu, as can be seen from these symptom descriptions, others will suffer much more. ***Since this is a book about homoeopathic treatment, I am only concentrating***

on the symptoms and modalities that you must look out for which will lead you to the homoeopathic remedy; I have avoided as much as I can any medical jargon or aspects which are only important from an allopathic (conventional) treatment's point of view.

In the Materia Medica and Repertory Sections of this book all the different aspects are covered. You should be prepared to follow through the developing symptoms from the initial fever and coldy symptoms, watching out for conjunctivitis, nose and/or gums bleeding, back and limb pains, gut problems or lung problems since they may soon appear. It would be quite normal to expect to start off with an initial fever remedy, such as Aconite, Baptisia, Belladonna, Oscillococcinum or Ferrum Phos. You would then move onto remedies to help limb pains/sensations, if they started to appear, such as Eup-perf., Baptisia, Lachesis, Pyrogen, Rhus Tox., Bryonia, Gelsemium or Merc.Sol. However, if the symptoms which next developed were digestive in nature, with vomiting and diarrhœa you might need to look at Carbo Veg., Nux Vomica, Ars.Alb., Kali Carb., Baptisia, Ipecac., Bryonia and others. If the symptoms go down to the lungs, starting with cough and chest pains, you would then be repertorizing for these and should be prepared to deal with pneumonia. Some of those with a very high fever may well develop encephalitis and become delirious, in which case you may be looking at remedies such as Belladonna, Aconite, Gelsemium, Baptisia and so on. Obviously, by being alert and dealing with each development as soon as it emerges, it would be most likely that many of the more serious types of Bird flu would be prevented entirely, or else they would be nipped in the bud so that they never seriously weaken or threaten the life of the patient. If the symptoms turn into the most severe, you would have the remedies and knowledge to treat the patient and get them fit and well again. The precautions outlined in Chapter Six on prevention should make it less likely that people would develop the more serious symptoms, but the information in this book will give you the ability to deal with all types of symptoms should they develop.

Taking the homœopathic case

When using homœopathic remedies you choose the remedy by the *individual symptoms that characterize a person's illness*, not the common symptoms which everyone may have with that particular disease. So you could have twenty people with measles and each of them will have a particular unique picture of symptoms which belong to them only, and some common symptoms which they all will have. It is the symptoms that are *unique* to the patient, which build up an *individual* picture, that *differentiate* that person from the other patients, which are important for choosing the similar remedy and *point to the right homœopathic remedy.*

In order to choose a homœopathic remedy you need to have a great deal of individual detail about the patient as a whole. You should consider each part of the body affected, so that you can work out what differentiates one patient from the next.

Here are some symptoms to get you started so you can build up a picture of the uniqueness of the individual. You should consider the following:-

Sore throats: You must find out if one side is worse; if it started on one side and moved to the other; what type of pain there is; where the pain travels to or if it stays in one place; whether warm water or cold water is less painful on the throat; and which is easier to swallow, food or drink. What colour is the throat and are there any ulcers on it? Use a torch to have a good look. Are they thirsty or not, and if they are, what do they want and how are they drinking it, sips, or fast by the glassful, or in any other manner?

Headaches: Do position, touch, pressure, noise, light, or movement affect the headache in any way? If so, in what way does it improve or worsen? Is it worse on one side, does it change side, does the room temperature or weather or air affect it? What does the face look like, is the colour different from usual? If the fever is very high, is there delirium, is the patient incoherent? If so, see 'Appearance and behaviour' below.

Back and limb pains: What is the pain like, is one side of the body worse than the other, do movement, touch or pressure affect the pain? Are the pains affecting the bones mostly, or the muscles mostly, and are there any other symptoms?

Eyes: Look for types of conjunctivitis since it is known to be a possible symptom of Bird flu. Is there a discharge, and, if so, is it bland, or acrid, thick or thin, watery or lumpy, green, cream, yellow, clear or changeable? Does light affect the eyes, what is the pain like or is it painless, and are the whites of the eyes discoloured in some way?

Fever, chill and sweat: Here you need to observe how the patient is during both the fever and the chill, as the reaction to external temperature may be different according to which they are suffering from at the time. So consider reactions to draughts, cool applications or hot applications, wanting the bedclothes on or off, and wanting the window open or shut. Look out for other weather reactions which could be affecting them, or which could have contributed to increasing their susceptibility to the disease; wet windy weather, cold windy weather, dry weather, hot summer, warm winter, cold winter, damp, wet or anything else. You must also consider whether sweat is bringing some relief or not. Is there a particular part of the body that is sweatier than the rest, or are they bone dry with no sweat, or do they have very smelly sweat?

Cough, chest and breathing: Have they any symptoms in this area yet, did they come on quickly or slowly, is the cough loose or dry, is expectoration easy or difficult, thick, thin, bloody, smelly, or what? What colour is the expectoration? What position is most comfortable for them, or worse for them, when they cough, or for their chest pain? What makes their breathing easier or more difficult? Which part of their chest hurts? How does the cough react to cold, warm, wet, cool air or to draughts? Does a drink help or not?

Appearance and behaviour: What does their skin look like, is the sweat bloody or not, what is the colour and smell and appearance of any discharge, whether from eyes, skin or lungs or rectum? Is their face a different colour from usual? Are they restless, does that make any pain worse or does it help? Are they lethargic and hardly moving, does keeping still help the pain? Does talking help? Do they want you there or are they happier being left alone? Do they want you there, but not want you to talk, or not want to have to talk to you? Are they cross and irritable, weepy, critical, oversensitive, fearful or showing any other particular emotion? Are they delirious? Are they restless, violent, comatose, loquacious or shrieking?

Digestive system: Here you must consider their likes and dislikes concerning both food and drink that are different from usual and what may make them feel better or worse. Also you must know if there are any abdominal pains, discomfort or distension. Is there any diarrhœa, if so you must find out what the stools are like and find out about any pains.

One very important point to make about taking the case and discovering the symptoms unique to the individual is that if anyone has been taking Tamiflu, Relenza or any other medication the individual symptoms will be less clear, sometimes may be completely hidden and it will be virtually impossible to see an accurate picture, to take a correct case or to treat anyone successfully.

Having given all the above symptoms some thought, write down all the symptoms which help build up a picture of the patient. You then re-write the list in order of importance of the symptoms.

Heirarchy of symptoms

As a general rule, any symptom that is very marked is very important. So severe nose bleeding with every cough would be more important than a very slight bloody nasal discharge just once. Profuse sweating without any relief, time and time again, would be more important than being rather damply sweaty some of the time. Violent and frequent diarrhœa would be more important than once only.

The more peculiar a symptom is the more important it becomes in the hierarchy. This means that feeling boiling hot yet wanting to be covered up is more important an indication in choosing a remedy than feeling boiling hot but wanting to be uncovered. Being icy cold but wanting cold air on your face is odder than being hot and wanting cool air. Being desperately hot with a high fever and having a dry mouth but without thirst, is more important than the same high fever with thirst. While *all* the unique individual symptoms are *very* important, the more *peculiar* they are, the *higher* they move up the hierarchical scale.

You also divide symptoms up into Mentals, Generals and Particulars. When choosing a remedy, any emotional symptoms (Mentals) are the most important. Symptoms which affect the whole of a person (rather than just a part of them) are called Generals, and are the next most important symptoms for choosing a remedy. These are the ones which a patient describes as "**I** am feeling cold, **I** am feeling sweaty,

I am better for fresh air". The next most important are the Particular symptoms which refer to just one bit of the patient. These are the ones the patient will describe as "**my** head is hurting, **my** throat is burning, **my** eyes are aching". So the patient might say "**I** am feeling icy cold and **my** feet are aching". The patient is feeling icy cold which affects all of him, and is therefore a General symptom, which is more important than his feet aching which is a Particular symptom, affecting only one part of him. So the order of importance is Mentals, then Generals, then Particulars. However, if any one of these symptoms is very, very intense, it would move up a rung in the hierarchical ladder. It may seem rather pernickety to analyze like this, but it becomes very important if you have to choose between two or three closely indicated remedies. It draws attention to the remedies covering the most important symptoms, making it much easier and quicker to select the remedy.

By and large the hierarchy of symptoms is common sense and it also matters more in long-term constitutional case taking where it becomes considerably more complicated. If you follow these rules you will be less likely to focus on one or two, possibly minor, symptoms only, and more likely to look at the patient **as a whole**.

Repertorization

Once you have taken the details of the case, you should take a copy of the Repertorization Chart at the end of this chapter and start filling it in. It is important to enter the name obviously, but the date as well as the time is important in a fast-moving acute disease. You should also number the chart so that you know which one you are referring to when you fill in the Patient Record (another blank form at end of this chapter). You enter your re-written symptom list in the appropriate hierarchical order. You do not necessarily need to fill in all ten symptom slots, but they are there should you need them; sometimes you may need more than that. Then you go through the Repertory in Section Two looking to see which remedies have the symptoms in the case and mark them off in the corresponding symptom/remedy box. This will build up a picture of the most indicated remedies on your Repertorization Chart. Having done that you then read through those remedies in the Materia Medica in Section Three and see which ones fit the picture best. The better and more clearly you have observed the symptoms and taken the case in the first place, the easier and simpler it will be to choose the homœopathic remedy. I must stress at this point that you **MUST** choose the remedy in this way. **DO NOT** read through the Materia Medica first, pick out a few symptoms and choose a remedy which appears to fit based on a few symptoms only. That way you will only find a partially similar remedy which will not work very well and the patient will most probably get much worse. You cannot risk making such a mistake and wasting time when treating such a potentially serious and fast moving condition as Bird flu. That way will lead to disaster and you must not do that with a possible life threatening and rapidly developing illness. I know that sometimes many of my patients have not repertorized but guessed the remedy instead, due to either laziness or impatience, and because the conditions they have been treating, despite being unpleasant, have not been very serious. You must take the case, then repertorize, and only having done that should you start looking through the most indicated remedies in the Materia Medica. If you do it methodically and look at the patient as a whole, you will be unlikely to make mistakes. You have to do it the correct way in a disease that could be life threatening. There may well be not much time, perhaps only a few days, and sometimes only few hours, in which to treat them; you must get it right from the start.

Chapter Four

Some Demonstration Cases

Case 1

The following case is an imaginary one to show exactly how repertorization is done.

You have a middle-aged person who is going down with a sore throat, slight head cold and a fever. The usual aches and pains which occur during flu have begun and he is developing an extremely dry, cough which started rapidly, within a few hours. It occurs mostly whenever he tries to talk. When he coughs he says it hurts his chest very badly with sharp pains. When you look at him his lips are dry and cracked and he is very thirsty for cold drinks. You are in a panic as you know Bird flu is now spreading fast and are afraid this could be it. His limbs hurt and generally he is complaining a lot and seems to be very irritable. He does not want the room warm and gets cross with you when you shut the window.

From the above, what rubrics are you going to choose? What rubrics are personal to him and are NOT the ones that are common to many flu conditions? Here is a list:

Travelling fast down to his lungs
Dry cough worse for talking
Dry lips
Very thirsty for cold drinks
Chest pains are sharp
Limbs hurt
Irritable
Worse for warmth
Better for cool air

Now you are going to rearrange the list in order of importance and intensity and also slightly re-word them to suit repertorization. This is what you should come up with:

Irritable: Emotional (Mental) symptoms are most important.
Warmth aggravates: This is a General symptom which affects the whole of him.
Cool ameliorates: This is another important General symptom.
Thirsty for cold drink: This is an intense General symptom in his case.
Cough worse for movement: This only applies to his chest, not the whole of him, so comes below the General symptoms but high up among the Particular symptoms because it is quite severe and is his main complaint.
Sharp chest pains: This is a very strong Particular symptom affecting his chest only.
Lips very dry: This also is a strong Particular symptom as his lips are so very dry and painful but it still only affects part of him.
Limbs hurt: This Particular symptom does not have much detail and at this stage seems less important than the others. It could become a more important feature if it were more intense and then it would probably be described with more detail.

So now let us fill out the Repertorization Chart and see if a clear remedy is indicated.

REPERTORIZATION CHART	NUMBER………
NAME:	DATE & TIME:
RUBRICS:	
1 Irritable	6 Lips very dry
2 Better cool air, worse warmth	7 Limbs painful
3 Thirst, very thirsty for cold	
4 Cough worse movement	
5 Sharp chest pains	

REMEDY NAME	1	2	3	4	5	6	7	8	9	10
Aconite		X	X							
Ant-tart.	X									
Apis										
Arg-nit.										
Ars-alb.			X		X					
Ars-iod.										
Baptisia						X				
Belladonna	X									
Bryonia	X	X	X	X	X	X				
Camphor			X							
Carb-ac.										
Carbo-veg.		X				X				
Chelidonium										
Crot-hor.										
Eup-perf.			X							
Ferr-phos.			X							
Gelsemium										
Hep-sulph.	X									
Ipecac.										
Kali-carb.					X					
Lachesis		X	X							
Merc-sol.			X							
Mur-ac.										
Nat-sulph.										
Nit-ac.	X					X				
Nux-v.	X									
Oscillococcinum										
Phosphorus			X							
Pulsatilla		X								
Pyrogen										
Rhus-tox.										
Sanguinaria		X								
Sulphur		X								
Verat-alb.										
Verat-vir.										

I have not filled in the seventh rubric remedies as there is not enough detail; I would need to know more about the type of pain before being able to fill that in properly. I have deliberately shown this, as patients finding it difficult to describe symptoms is the kind of thing that happens during real case taking.

Obviously the remedy in this case is Bryonia and I made it easy for a first venture into repertorizing, so that you can get the general idea as to what one is supposed to do. Now, suppose there had not been such a clear remedy indicated and perhaps Eup-perf. was about equally indicated alongside Bryonia. Then one would have to look at the patient again and see if there were any symptoms that had been missed, and if there had been, add them in to see if they made a greater emphasis on one or other remedy. If there were no missed symptoms, you would then look up both remedies in the Materia Medica and see which seemed to fit the patient best as a whole. In an acute serious disease one remedy is usually strongly indicated because the symptoms are much clearer the more serious the condition is. In acutes which are not particularly serious it is often puzzling which remedy to choose because there is no obvious remedy indicated (perhaps the patient needs no treatment at that time) but with Bird flu it will probably be both clear and easy. The main thing to be sure about is that you have taken the case thoroughly and well, and have not missed anything.

Another scenario could be that you had all the symptoms indicating Bryonia to be the remedy, but the patient actually by then had pneumonia, and it was obvious from the location of the pains that the patient's lungs were affected on the left side, whereas Bryonia is most indicated for the right lung. In such a case you should double check that none of the left lung remedies (Acon., Calc.Carb., Lach., Nat.Sulph., Phos., or Sanguinaria) was not more indicated **as a whole**. If not, which would show up in the repertorization, you would still give Bryonia because the picture **as a whole** fits Bryonia much more than any other remedy. One is always trying to choose the most similar remedy, it cannot necessarily be exact. This is where the hierarchy of symptoms becomes crucial, and the reason why it is necessary to fill in the chart starting with the most important symptoms, with the least important coming up last. That way you can always see at a glance, when two or three remedies might be running neck and neck, which one is more important; you would choose the remedy with the most similar earlier rubrics (perhaps numbers 1-4) rather than the remedy with the most similar later rubrics (perhaps numbers 6-10). Also, you would check this out in the Materia Medica by reading up the remedies concerned, to be sure you had chosen correctly.

Case 2

Here is another example to try.

A four year old child with a very loose sounding cough but expectoration was almost impossible to raise. However, it sounded as though it should be easy to raise because it was so loose and rattling. He had to sit up to cough. The patient was extremely sweaty, running a fever and very tired and weak. He seemed to be worse round 3 am. He was feeling sick but had not actually vomited. He was not thirsty at all whether during the fever or in the chill, but when he did try to drink anything it hurt his throat. His face had a bluey tinge round the mouth area. He had a headache on the right side, but it was not very severe.

Here are the rubrics you would choose from the above case taking:-
Loose cough, rattling in lungs
Difficult expectoration
Sits up to cough
Generally sweaty and feverish
Worse 3 am
Nausea
Thirstless
Discolouration on face, bluey tinge
Worse right side

You would then re-write the list. First of all you would notice that there appear to be no Mentals recorded so you would start with the Generals which would be the time aggravation at 3 am, the thirstlessness and the right sidedness. However, there is only one right sided symptom, nor is it severe, which makes the General symptom of right sidedness less strongly indicated; it should go lower down in the hierarchical list, despite it being a General symptom. The cough is very severe and intense so this Particular symptom and the symptoms concerning it are more important than the other Particular symptom, the mild headache. The new list would look like this:

Worse at 3 am: A General symptom.
Thirstlessness: A General symptom.
Loose cough with difficult expectoration: This is important as you would expect a loose cough to have easy expectoration, so this is a strong Particular symptom.
Sits up to cough: A Particular symptom.
Blue round mouth: A Particular symptom.
Worse right side: A General symptom but not a very intense symptom compared to the other Particular symptoms above.

I have left out the nausea, sweat and fever because at this stage there are not any unique details that would make them special for the patient. Should greater detail emerge, I would include them at once later on. However, you should bear these symptoms in mind when checking through the Materia Medica.

REPERTORIZATION CHART			NUMBER...........							
NAME:			DATE & TIME:							
RUBRICS:										
1 Worse at 3am		6 Blue round mouth								
2 Thirstless		7 Worse right side								
3 Difficult expectoration		8								
4 Loose cough		9								
5 Must sit up to cough		10								
REMEDY NAME	1	2	3	4	5	6	7	8	9	10
Aconite										
Ant-tart.		X	X	X	X	X				
Apis		X					X			
Arg-nit.										
Ars-alb.					X					
Ars-iod.			X							
Baptisia										
Belladonna	X						X			
Bryonia					X					
Camphor						X				
Carb-ac.										
Carbo-veg.				X		X				
Chelidonium			X	X			X			
Crot-hor.							X			
Eup-perf.				X						
Ferr-phos.										
Gelsemium		X								
Hep-sulph.				X	X					
Ipecac.		X	X	X						
Kali-carb.	X		X	X						
Lachesis										
Merc-sol.							X			
Mur-ac.										
Nat-sulph.				X						
Nit-ac.										
Nux-v.	X									
Oscillococcinum				X						
Phosphorus										
Pulsatilla		X		X	X					
Pyrogen					X					
Rhus-tox.										
Sanguinaria	X		X	X			X			
Sulphur				X						
Verat-alb.				X		X				
Verat-vir.										

Looking at the above repertorization chart there is only one remedy, Ant.Tart., which has five of the six important symptoms covered, so that is the most likely remedy, but we should also have a look at Sang. because that has four rubrics and one of these is an important General symptom, worse at 3 am. However, if we look further, one of its four rubrics is the least important so we should take that into consideration as well. When you read up the two remedies in the Materia Medica you will see that this case has none of the congestion and redness that Sanguinaria has throughout its remedy picture, but it does have the bluey look round the mouth of Ant.Tart. Reading Ant.Tart. you will also notice that it is particularly useful for the very old and young, and this patient is four years old. This is an additional reason for Ant.Tart. which has not been repertorized so it adds weight to the correct choice being Ant.Tart.

One reason I have used this case as a demonstration case, is that it has two strong Belladonna symptoms. Anyone with a very little basic knowledge of homœopathy could easily latch onto these Belladonna symptoms, and if they did not bother to repertorize the case properly they could in their impatience, fear, or hurry, think Belladonna to be the remedy. Obviously it is not because Belladonna has a dry cough, none of the loose rattle in the lungs, no blue or grey discolouration of the face and would be totally the wrong remedy. Again, if someone has slight knowledge of homœopathy they could perhaps think Pulsatilla to be the remedy as it has a loose cough and has to sit up to cough. Again that would be wrong as Pulsatilla has a loose cough which not only has very easy expectoration but also is often drier at night. A strong Pulsatilla symptom is that their coughs are always worse in a stuffy warm room, but this is not even mentioned in the case, so that would be yet another reason for Pulsatilla not to be the remedy. So here you can see the importance of repertorizing, not being impatient, and working it out correctly. People who are used to cutting corners and not taking a proper case, nor doing a repertorization, are the ones who might choose Belladonna or Pulsatilla. They will be wasting precious time, which although may be available in ordinary flu is NOT available with Bird flu. Their laziness could result in a death.

Case 3

Here is another demonstration case.

A 30 year old man arrived home from work with a headache and a runny nose and was generally feeling under the weather. He woke up in the morning with violent aching and soreness in his limbs and back and felt freezing cold. He was feeling very sick as well and could not stand even the thought of eating breakfast. The violent headache was worse if he lay down and the worst pain was at the back of the head. He was shivering with cold. He said any movement made the aches and pains much worse as if the bones were broken. He wanted to be kept warm and was worse if the window was open.

The following rubrics are the ones you would choose from the above picture:

Worse in the morning (this is the time when the symptoms became really bad)
Pains, aching and soreness in limbs, as if bones broken
Violent pains in his back, aching and soreness
Worse for movement
Headache worse in the occiput area, the back of his head
Headache worse lying down
Headache worse for pressure (it could be either the position of lying down which makes his headache worse or the pressure of the head against the pillow, or both of these)
Shivering and chills with the pains
Worse for cold air (he wanted the window closed)
Better if covered up during the chill
The thought of food made him feel sick

You would rearrange the rubrics in order of importance. No emotional symptoms are recorded so you would start with the General ones and the more intense Particular ones.

Intense aching and soreness of his back: While this is a Particular symptom only, it becomes more important because this is a very intense pain and the main symptom that is bothering him; it is the one that was bad enough to wake him up. It also covers not just the back but the limbs as well; ie it is affecting more of him than just his back, so with both Particular areas affected it almost becomes a General.
Intense aching and soreness of his limbs, as if the bones were broken: See first reason.
Worse in the morning: A General symptom.
Worse for movement: This is a General symptom and applies to the most intensely painful symptom that he has.
Shivering with the chills, feeling it mostly in his back: This is a General symptom and applies to all of him, although it is worse in his back.
Worse for cold air: Another General symptom.
The thought of food makes him feel sick: Again this is a General symptom.
Headache affecting the back of his head mostly: This is a Particular symptom.
Headache worse lying down: A Particular symptom.
Headache worse for pressure: A Particular symptom.

Having re-written the rubric list in order of importance you must now fill in the Repertorization Chart.

REPERTORIZATION CHART	NUMBER………
NAME:	DATE & TIME:
RUBRICS:	
1 Pain in back, aching, soreness	6 Worse cold air
2 Pain in limbs, as if bones broken	7 Nausea, worse at thought of food
3 Worse in morning, first thing	8 Headache in the occiput area
4 Worse for movement	9 Headache worse lying down
5 Shivering chills, generally & in the back	10

REMEDY NAME	1	2	3	4	5	6	7	8	9	10
Aconite			X							
Ant-tart.				X						
Apis			X							
Arg-nit.										
Ars-alb.							X			
Ars-iod.										
Baptisia			X							
Belladonna				X					X	
Bryonia				X						
Camphor								X		
Carb-ac.										
Carbo-veg.										
Chelidonium				X						
Crot-hor.										
Eup-perf.	X	X	X	X	X	X	X	X	X	
Ferr-phos.										
Gelsemium	X			X	X			X	X	
Hep-sulph.						X				
Ipecac.							X			
Kali-carb.										
Lachesis			X							
Merc-sol.						X				
Mur-ac.										
Nat-sulph.										
Nit-ac.						X				
Nux-v.				X		X				
Oscillococcinum										
Phosphorus								X		
Pulsatilla										
Pyrogen						X				
Rhus-tox.	X					X		X		
Sanguinaria								X		
Sulphur										
Verat-alb.						X				
Verat-vir.								X		

I want to comment on the choice of rubrics. With the first rubric, the patient might actually have said "My back is agony, it is really hurting badly", and, however hard you tried to make him be more exact in his description, you may not have been able to get any further details. This is the sort of thing that happens when taking a real case and can be very frustrating. When you look this up in order to choose the correct rubrics, you would find various descriptions under the heading "Back". It would seem from the patient's description that he cannot say whether or not it is the bones or muscles that are hurting, so in this case you would combine the various rubrics to make sure you covered all the remedies. You would combine, Back, muscular soreness, Back, broken feeling, aching bones, and Back, generally stiff, particularly lower back. These three rubrics cover all the possibilities, there is no point including other rubrics for lower back only, but choose the ones that cover the whole back.

The second rubric is much easier because he is referring to his limbs and says it feels as if the bones are broken. Here he actually mentions the bones in preference to the muscles being sore so it is easy to choose Extremities, aching soreness as if bones broken.

For the third rubric you need to look up under Time/Speed, and you will find Time/Speed, worse in the early morning, Time/Speed, worse 7-9 am and Time/Speed, worse on waking. From the symptom description, the rubrics Time/Speed, worse 7-9 am and Time/Speed, worse on waking would be the ones to choose. I feel his symptoms would have had to begin much earlier to use the rubric Time/Speed, worse in the early morning.

The fourth rubric is straightforward, Position/Motion, worse for motion.

The fifth you find under Weather, Body Temperature, Reactions to, chills in the back and shivering.

The remaining rubrics are straightforward but I have left out the last one because it is not really clear whether his headache is worse for pressure or not. This is something that could become more obvious later on, or it could disappear as a symptom completely.

The choice of remedy for this case would clearly be Eup-perf. at this stage. However, one of the reasons I chose this description is because I know that many people with a just a little homœopathic knowledge may well notice that there are many well known Gelsemium symptoms in it. Those who are too rushed to take the case thoroughly or to repertorize properly, could easily think it could be either Gelsemium or Eup-perf. and choose Gelsemium in error. When done correctly it is **obviously** Eup-perf. as it fits totally, whereas Gelsemium fits only partially. There is no time to make that kind of mistake with Bird flu.

Case 4

Here is one last sample case. It would be a good idea if you did not read the repertorization but tried to work it out for yourself to see how you get on.

A middle-aged woman went down with flu symptoms very quickly and within a few hours had a raging fever, very dry parched mouth and slight thirst, very smelly breath, some mouth ulcers and very smelly sweat. The stools were bloody, her back was aching slightly and she could not get her breath easily; the difficulty in breathing was quite a strong symptom. She wanted fresh air, and her skin was taking on a purply bluey red colour, particularly on her face. She could hardly talk or tell her symptoms in her confusion and misery.

The rubrics chosen were:
Fast onset
Smelly generally, breath and sweat
Stools bloody
Difficulty breathing
Desire for fresh air
Purply bluey red discolouration to the face
Confused, could hardly talk, muddled
Dry parched mouth

Rearranged in order of importance the list would look like this:
Confusion, can hardly talk, muddled: This is the only Mental symptom.
Very smelly discharges: This is a General symptom.
Desire for fresh air: This is a General symptom.
Difficulty breathing: This is a General symptom.
Sweat smelly: This is a General symptom.
Sudden onset: This is a General symptom.
Breath smelly: This is a Particular symptom.
Stools bloody: This is a Particular symptom.
Dry parched mouth: This is a Particular symptom.
Face purply bluey red colour: This is a Particular symptom.

I have left out the "some thirst" symptom because it is neither very strong nor is there no thirst. If either of these were the case it would be much more significant and one should be observant and notice if the symptom changed.

REPERTORIZATION CHART			NUMBER………							
NAME:			DATE & TIME:							
RUBRICS:										
1 Confusion			6 Sudden onset							
2 Discharges generally smelly			7 Stools bloody							
3 Desire for fresh air			8 Mouth, breath smelly							
4 Difficulty breathing			9 Very dry parched mouth							
5 Sweat smelly			10 Face purply bluey red							
REMEDY NAME	1	2	3	4	5	6	7	8	9	10
Aconite				X		X				
Ant-tart.				X			X			
Apis				X		X				
Arg-nit.										
Ars-alb.		X	X	X				X		
Ars-iod.			X							
Baptisia	X	X	X	X	X	X	X	X	X	X
Belladonna						X				
Bryonia	X								X	
Camphor										
Carb-ac.		X				X		X		
Carbo-veg.		X	X					X		
Chelidonium								X		
Crot-hor.	X	X			X		X	X		
Eup-perf.				X						
Ferr-phos.						X				
Gelsemium				X						
Hep-sulph.		X								
Ipecac.			X				X			
Kali-carb.										
Lachesis	X			X			X	X		X
Merc-sol.		X		X	X		X	X		
Mur-ac.								X		
Nat-sulph.										
Nit-ac.		X		X	X					
Nux-v.				X				X		
Oscillococcinum										
Phosphorus				X		X	X			
Pulsatilla			X	X						
Pyrogen		X			X			X		
Rhus-tox.										
Sanguinaria	X			X						
Sulphur		X								
Verat-alb.										
Verat-vir.										

Choosing the rubrics is fairly easy for this case. You could perhaps have added in the rubric "early stages" as it was still early on, and you could also have added in the backache, but it was not a very strong symptom. The General symptoms (numbers 2, 3, 4, 5 and 6) were all fairly equally indicated, except for the degree of smelliness which was much stronger. The Particular symptoms were all fairly equal in importance, but the bloody stools were probably the most serious; the intensity of the dry mouth was very strong, as well as the smelliness of the breath being important because smelliness ran throughout the whole symptom picture.

It is obvious that the homœopathic remedy in this case is Baptisia, particularly when you read up the Baptisia description in the Materia Medica. However, if this case had not been repertorized properly the remedies Lachesis, Merc.Sol. and possibly Ars.Alb. might have come to mind as well as Baptisia. They are all well known for smelly discharges: Lachesis also for the purply discolouration and breathing difficulties; Ars.Alb. for the smelly discharges and breathing difficulties; and Merc.Sol. for the bloody stools with the smelly discharges. Again this case demonstrates the importance of taking the case properly first, then repertorizing it, and only after that, looking up the most indicated remedies in the Materia Medica.

Comparison of some remedies

In order to help you get to know the remedies better, and become familiar with the kind of differences between them which are important, I am now going to compare some remedies which initially might appear to have very similar symptoms, but on closer study are in fact very different.

First we are going to look at some very cold remedies. The ones I have chosen are Carbo Veg., Camphor and Veratrum Alb. All three remedies are icy cold, blue with cold and you would never give any of these remedies if there were not coldness in the patient's symptom picture. However, despite being so cold both Camphor and Carbo Veg. want even more cold, in so far as Camphor does not want to be covered up and desires cold drinks, and Carbo Veg. wants fresh cool air and fanning. Veratrum Alb., although being worse for cold food and drink, has a cough that gets worse on going into a warm room. Just to be contrary Camphor does not want to be covered up except during the high fever. While all three remedies are in a state of collapse, Camphor may have a persistent nosebleed, Carbo Veg. has particularly smelly discharges and may ooze dark blood and Veratrum Album has copious violent vomiting, purging, diarrhœa and sweats. Despite being exhausted, Veratrum Alb. is the most energetic of the three simply because of the violence of the vomiting and diarrhœa; Veratrum Alb. is terribly weak in between times. Veratrum Alb. and Carbo Veg. can both have rattling mucus in the lungs, but Camphor does not. Carbo Veg. has an enormously distended abdomen with wind, burping and colic while Veratrum Alb. has all the vomiting and purging. So while you might start off thinking these three remedies to be fairly similar since they all have such icy cold symptoms, in fact you could never confuse them as there are so many other ways to differentiate them. You could also compare all three remedies to Ars.Alb. which is another chilly remedy, but Ars.Alb. has burning pains which are ameliorated by heat. Carbo Veg. also has burning pains but they are not ameliorated by heat. It also is better for fresh cool air like Ars.Alb. Ars.Alb. can also be extremely restless, despite its exhaustion and collapsed state, but Carbo Veg. is in a state of collapse and is too weak to move.

You could then compare some remedies which have a lot of haemorrhaging in their remedy picture, such as Phos., Ipecac., Carbo Veg., Lachesis, and Crotalus Horridus. Both Phos. and Ipecac. bleed rather bright red blood, while Ipecac's haemorrhaging is often gushing, and both can be profuse. Carbo Veg. oozes blood which is rather dark in colour, Lachesis bleeds rather thin blood with bits in it rather like straw and Crotalus Horridus bleeds very dark blood, which can almost seem as though it is black. Crotalus Horr. bleeds so much that it even comes through the pores of the skin as well as from any orifice of the body. From these descriptions you can see that just looking at the type of blood and bleeding alone you can tell the difference between these remedies, before you even begin to look at the rest of the symptom picture.

At the beginning of the Repertory there are details about how it works and how to find the rubric you are looking for. You can use it to find all the remedies which have bleeding as part of their symptom picture, all the remedies which have strong one-sidedness, all the remedies' different types of discharges, all the remedies with various reactions to cold or heat, all the remedies with strong time aggravations and so on.

I hope this makes you realize how very important it is to take the case thoroughly, repertorize it properly and choose the remedy as a result of good case taking and repertorization, rather than a random panicky choice from dipping into the Materia Medica. It will not take long to do it correctly, and however serious Bird flu may become, there is ALWAYS time to spend a few minutes working it out properly. It is also a very good idea to note down how the patient responds to each dose of remedy by keeping a good time and symptom response sheet. This will help you during the few hours or days you will be looking after them and prescribing for them. You should photocopy the Patient Record and the Repertorization Chart on the following pages so that you have plenty of copies, bearing in mind you might end up helping quite a few people.

PATIENT RECORD:			NAME:
Date & Time	Remedy & Potency	Rep No.	Response Details

REPERTORIZATION CHART	NUMBER.........
NAME:	DATE & TIME:
RUBRICS:	
1	6
2	7
3	8
4	9
5	10

REMEDY NAME	1	2	3	4	5	6	7	8	9	10
Aconite										
Ant-tart.										
Apis										
Arg-nit.										
Ars-alb.										
Ars-iod.										
Baptisia										
Belladonna										
Bryonia										
Camphor										
Carb-ac.										
Carbo-veg.										
Chelidonium										
Crot-hor.										
Eup-perf.										
Ferr-phos.										
Gelsemium										
Hepar-sulph.										
Ipecac.										
Kali-carb.										
Lachesis										
Merc-sol.										
Mur-ac.										
Nat-sulph.										
Nit-ac.										
Nux-v.										
Oscillococcinum										
Phosphorus										
Pulsatilla										
Pyrogen										
Rhus-tox.										
Sanguinaria										
Sulphur										
Verat-alb.										
Verat-vir.										

Chapter Five

Prescribing the remedies and the size of the dose

One dose is always one pill, one pilule or 1-3 drops of liquid remedy. The quantity does not matter, but the frequency of the dosage matters considerably. The remedy stimulates your immune system into some action to push out the disease. It is the frequency of these doses, or stimulations to heal, that matters, not the amount of remedy given. It would have the same effect if you took one pill or 20 at a time, but it would be rather a waste of the 19 pills you did not need.

Frequency of prescribing remedies

Once you have chosen the remedy for the stage of Bird flu which you are treating, you then have to decide on the potency and frequency of prescribing. As far as frequency of the dose is concerned you have to remember that **the remedy's job is to kick-start the immune system to begin to heal itself and thus enable the body to throw off the disease. Initially you give the remedy in a 30, repeating it every 10 to 30 minutes or so until you get a response and a sign of improvement.**

Signs of improvement:
The patient falls into a peaceful sleep.
The patient feels and looks improved, and the symptoms have become less painful and less severe.
The patient feels better although the symptoms are still there; that means that he is better in himself but still has all the symptoms. The pain may be as bad but the patient is coping better with it.
The patient vomits and feels better afterwards.

When any of these signs of improvement occur they may last for virtually any length of time; it could be simply a few minutes or a few hours or more. Once the remedy has stimulated the body into starting to improve, the body takes over the healing process; you do not need to give any more remedy until the improvement ceases. You may find you will be giving the remedy very frequently, or at long or varied intervals, because you only repeat it whenever the patient relapses.

Signs of relapsing:

Symptoms which had calmed down or disappeared, reappear.
Pain and discomfort return.
The improvement seems to have reached a plateau and there is no more progress for the better.

When any of these relapsing signs recur you repeat the remedy until improvement sets in again. If improvement does not happen you would go up in potency. In an acute situation, generally speaking you should repeat the remedy for about an hour or so (unless the patient is going downhill fast), and if there really is no change at all when you go through the list of "Signs of Improvement" (above) you would go up in potency. On the next higher potency you would repeat the remedy as above until improvement sets in. As soon as improvement has begun, you stop the remedy, because when that happens it means that the patient's immune system has begun to work properly and has taken over the healing, so you need not give any more remedy; you only repeat it when the patient starts to relapse. Often initial response will occur after only very few doses (anything from one to four doses) but repetition could be needed every five to ten minutes, for as long as an hour or even more, before the patient becomes significantly better. As the patient improves the intervals between doses should begin to lengthen. If repetition is required one to four hourly, or at even longer intervals, and progress is continuing, it would be considered to be going very well. During such times there could be the odd relapse when you may suddenly have to repeat the remedy much more frequently, or go up in potency; always repeat it more frequently first and only go up in potency if that does not work.

You carry on in this way until the patient is better, always being on the look-out for changes in the symptoms, which may indicate that you should do a further repertorization to check that you have the most similar remedy. **Do not change the remedy, even if the symptoms have changed, providing the remedy is still working. You only change the remedy if the symptoms have changed and the patient has stopped improving.**

Choosing the potency

- Ideally start with the remedy in a 30.
- You would go up to a 200 if you felt that there was no improvement, or only slight improvement from the 30.
- If you felt that the 200 was not helping enough you would go to a 1M if the person was either elderly or weak or both. You would skip the 1M and go straight to the 10M if the patient was being energetically ill, was very fit normally, was young not old, was delirious and/or some of the symptoms were affecting the emotional level.

- If you were giving a 1M and needed to go up in potency you would go up to a 10M next.
- If you need to go up from a 10M the next potency would be 50M, after the 50M it would be CM and after CM it would be MM.

In nearly all cases the potency needed will not be above a 30 or a 200. You just need to be aware that higher potencies are required sometimes, and these could be 1M, 10M, 50M, CM or MM. Mostly in my practice in acute conditions I do not have to go above a 200. However, there are occasions when a 1M or a 10M is required, and much less frequently I have to go even higher.

Some other important rules on potencies and prescribing

- Do not go to a higher potency unless you are sure the patient needs it. Higher is not better or more efficient with homœopathy, it is simply different. You have to match the energy of the patient to the potency of the remedy. If someone is delirious and throwing themselves around in the bed, or has very violent vomiting and diarrhœa, or is energetically bad tempered and abusive, or in any way seems to be showing a great deal of energy while they are ill, then the chances are you will need to go up to a higher potency sooner or later. However, do not be impatient or fearful, repeat the potency you are on a number of times, perhaps every five or ten minutes, for anything up to an hour, before going up. Over the years I have seen really extremely serious acute illnesses respond to very low potencies as well as others needing to up beyond a 10M or even a 50M.
- **Never go down in potency in the same remedy as this can aggravate the condition** which would be the last thing you would want to happen. If you are on a potency that is working, stay on it and do **not** go down; if they are improving, obviously you do not need to repeat the remedy until they relapse.
- If you need to change to a different remedy then of course you should start that new remedy lower, probably in a 30. However, if you find you are with a patient who appears to be responding mostly to high potencies it would be perfectly reasonable to go up in potency rather quicker than usual, if there had not been much response initially to the 30 in the new remedy.
- If a patient is very weak and feeble, has virtually no energy and perhaps can hardly talk, you would start on a 30 and may well find that is all you need. However, some people can be contrary and very occasionally in such a situation you will find you have to go up in potency to get a response. In such a situation check your case taking first to make sure you have left out nothing important, check your hierarchy of symptoms and your repertorization, and check the Materia Medica to make sure you are on the right remedy, then by all means go up if you are sure you are right.
- Remember that the wrong remedy will do nothing, it will not make the patient worse. If they seem to be getting worse on it, it is because giving the wrong remedy

(or the wrong potency) is like giving them no remedy at all, and their condition is simply deteriorating.
- A partially similar remedy will make a slight but inadequate improvement and if this has happened you should start again and find the right remedy.
- Do not get worked up about the idea that "with homœopathy you have to have an aggravation before you get better". This very occasionally happens with long-term chronic constitutional treatment, and is usually as a result of a healthy immune system pushing out toxins. In an acute, if such a thing occurs, it is so quick that unless you are an experienced homœopath no one will notice it at all, moreover it usually does not happen. I just mention this in passing as sometimes people get completely obsessed with the idea and have not really understood what is actually happening.
- Finally, do not, through impatience or fear (in both yourself as well as the patient), go up in potency too quickly, change the remedy too soon or stop following the hierarchy of symptoms. Always check the signs of improvement and signs of relapsing before making a decision, always check your case taking, repertorization and the Materia Medica first. As I say elsewhere in this book, it would be a good idea to become familiar with using homœopathy for other conditions such as those covered in the book *Homœopathy: The Modern Prescriber*, before attempting to treat Bird flu. It would help if you were able to contact your homœopath for extra guidance and support.

Plussing a remedy

This is a very useful way of making a remedy go further if your supplies are getting low. It is also a way of going up in potency in a gentle way if you do not have the next higher potency, or if you feel uncertain whether or not you should go up to the next higher potency. This is often the case when someone has been doing very well, or fairly well on a particular potency, but seems to have reached a plateau.

To do this you need a bottle, preferably of brown glass to protect the remedy from sunlight, but anything will do in an emergency. It should be 50-100 ml size, and it must be totally clean, without any residue of anything in it, particularly washing up liquid. Label the bottle with the original potency and date. (Do not use the glass bottle for any other remedy subsequently, unless you first carry out a very thorough sterilization in boiling water and then leave it to dry naturally, or in a very very low oven. Do not use any kind of washing up liquid to clean it either. When sterilizing the cap you must do it much more quickly or it will distort, and of course it must not go in the oven.) Put in a teaspoon of brandy or vodka to act as a preservative, fill it to the shoulders with either boiled then cooled water, or filtered water, and add about five pills of the remedy. Once the remedy pilules have dissolved, a dose is a dessertspoonful of the remedy. You hold it in the mouth, for approximately one minute before swallowing, as it works in your saliva in the usual way. However, after you have taken your first dose, and after all subsequent doses, you then replace that quantity of water, that is a dessertspoonful, into the bottle. This means that the level of water in the bottle never goes down. Before the next dose and every subsequent dose you must succuss the bottle a minimum of 12 times. This literally means banging the bottle fairly hard and firmly into the palm of your hand, or onto a book, 12 times. By this method you are diluting and succussing the remedy between each dose which actually makes it slightly more energetic, efficient and more curative. It is extraordinary how much difference this can make to help someone get better. This method never actually enables you to get to the next potency in the series, say from a 30C to exactly a 31C, but it seems to go off at a tangent of 30++++, in as many tiny little plussing stages as you need.

You can also plus a remedy in a glass of water. The succussing is not as efficient this way because even hearty stirring of the mixture in the glass is never as good as shaking it in a bottle. Also you need to cover the glass so that nothing else goes in it by mistake, as well as to try to keep it away from sunlight. However, if in a hurry, and maybe for just a short time, it is a useful way of doing it.

General nursing care when using homœopathy

Unfortunately these days people are not often used to nursing people but with Bird flu you will have to do so. When using homœopathic remedies there are a few extra things to be aware of. One is that if someone is very hot with a fever, the usual thing to do is to sponge them down with cool water. This is actually not at all a good idea when using homœopathy. First, if they are that hot and the fever is not coming down you need to give the remedy more frequently, or in a higher potency, so that the sponging should not be necessary. Second, if the remedy picture indicates Belladonna or any other remedy that is worse for cold wet applications and/or weather, sponging them down will actually make them much worse and in effect appears to antidote the remedy. Leave off the sponging and give more frequent doses, or a higher potency, of Belladonna or other indicated remedy. If someone wants darkness or hates bright light, close the curtains and switch off the light and do what they want. If they want the window wide open and cool air coming in, let them have it. Never know best, because their desires will lead you to clearer symptoms for case taking, and to the homœopathic remedy that will cure them. You could miss out on the symptoms which are important for choosing the remedy if you boss them around, and tell them what to do. Instead you should be calmly observing and noting their symptoms. There is of course a slight problem if they want to be in darkness, because you need to be able to see what they look like, what their appearance is, what their sweats are like, what their colour is, what position they want to be in, in what manner they drink any drinks, and so on. In this case you will *have* to have some light to get the right information but having done so, you should put things back how they want it to be.

Chapter Six

Homœopathic prevention of Bird flu

There are a number of different ways to prevent one catching Bird flu, or to reduce its severity, and many different opinions as to which is the best method. I will outline here the ones which I think should be best. First, and most important of all, is that you should have regular constitutional homœopathic treatment from a qualified homœopath so that any underlying illnesses or conditions that you may have, or have a tendency to have, are reduced or cured, enabling you to be as healthy as you can be. This also means trying to have genuine cures so that you are no longer dependant on conventional drugs, if that is at all possible; by doing so you will then be able to give homœopathic prevention and treatment the best chance of success. **Although homœopathic remedies cannot affect conventional drugs, conventional drugs usually make homœopathic remedies less efficient, and obscure the individual's picture.**

As soon as it is known that Bird flu has mutated and is being spread from human to human, the initial sequence of preventative remedies that should be taken is as follows:

1. Influenzinum 30 every morning and evening for four days in a row.
2. Then you should take the *Influenzinum 30 twice a day on one day every two weeks*. A good plan is to take it on alternate Sundays, starting on the first Sunday after completing No 1 above. You should also take *Bacillinum 30 twice a day on one day a month*. The best day to start this would be the Sunday after your first Sunday on Influenzinum 30. You should also take *Pneumococcus 30 twice a day on one day a month*. The best day for this would be the Sunday after your second Sunday on Influenzinum 30.

This means that having completed No 1 above, the prescribing at this stage for No 2 above, would look like this:-

First Sunday: Influenzinum 30 morning and evening.

Second Sunday: Bacillinum 30 morning and evening.

Third Sunday: Influenzinum 30 morning and evening.

Fourth Sunday: Pneumococcus 30 morning and evening.

You then would go back to the beginning of this sequence and repeat it as long as there remains a considerable risk.

However, the risk should reduce in time and there should be no need to continue like this month after month for various reasons. First, the pandemic may just possibly turn out to be not as serious as anticipated, in which case the frequency of the above remedies could be decreased. If this is the case you should double the intervals between each remedy date planned above. That would mean taking Influenzinum 30 on one day every month, Bacillinum 30 on one day every two months, and Pneumococcus 30 on one day every two months. Second, the pandemic will in time burn itself out so that much less prevention will be required. Third, you may catch it (but this would be a milder attack because of the prevention you will have undertaken) and having had it you will have gained immunity to it; in which case there will be no need for any more prevention. Finally, at some stage, hopefully within the first few months, a homœopathic pharmacy may have made a nosode of Bird flu; a nosode is a homœopathic remedy made from a disease product obtained from a person with the specific disease. This is assuming that there will still be some kind of postal service, so that you can be sent the remedy enabling you to take Bird flu nosode 30 as your prevention remedy, instead of the pattern of prescribing as described above. Also, further on in this chapter I describe how you can make up your own nosode of Bird flu, which you could use instead.

Another way to prevent the body from destroying itself is for homœopaths to prescribe the occasional dose of Lueticum 30 if they feel their patient needs it. Tuberculinum is also an excellent remedy for long-term prevention of over-reactions by running too high fevers, and is complementary to Lueticum. It is very similar to Bacillinum but has greater emphasis on dealing with the tendency for fevers going much too high. If your homœopath thinks taking some Lueticum 30 or Tuberculinum 30 occasionally is a good idea, you could add them into the prevention programme mentioned previously so that it would now look like this:-

First Sunday: Influenzinum 30, morning and evening
Second Sunday: Bacillinum 30, morning and evening
Third Sunday: Influenzinum 30, morning and evening
Fourth Sunday: Pneumococcus 30, morning and evening
Fifth Sunday: Influenzinum 30, morning and evening
Sixth Sunday: Tuberculinum 30, morning and evening
Seventh Sunday: Influenzinum 30, morning and evening
Eighth Sunday: Lueticum 30, morning and evening
then start the sequence again from the beginning.

As the risk becomes less you would eventually start taking the above at less frequent intervals; first changing from weekly doses in the above sequence to two weekly doses, then perhaps monthly doses.

You will find many other homœopathic recommendations for taking the above remedies which usually involve taking two or three of them mixed up in the same pill. While this is all right, homœopathic remedies actually work much better if taken separately, which is the reason I think alternating them is best. It is important, however, to remember that constitutional homœopathic treatment on a regular basis is the best method of all to keep you healthy.

Making a nosode out of Bird flu

If homœopathic pharmacies have been unable to make a Bird flu nosode, or if they have been able to, but there is no postal service to send it to you, it is possible to make one up yourself. Many people will not want to do this, but if you can, you will provide yourself with the best homœopathic prevention against Bird flu. **I must emphasize that you would be undertaking this at your own risk because it does mean close contact with the disease so you should follow the advice later on in this chapter about protective clothing; it is found under the heading of Practical Preparations and is very important as you should be extremely careful when making such a nosode.** However, if you have already had Bird flu you will be immune and need not worry about contact. There are quite a few different ways of doing this but I am going to describe the simplest and quickest.

Once you have put on the relevant protective clothing, you obtain some sputum from the sick person who has Bird flu. You only need a small amount, just one drop, but most people will find it too hard to believe that that could be enough; suffice it to say that quarter of a teaspoonful is fine, and more than you need. Put this in a brown glass bottle, a 100 ml size would be best, but in fact any type of bottle will do; it must be totally clean and without any soap residue in it. You fill it up at least two thirds full with water, personally I think it is better if it is filtered water but it does not have to be, and also I prefer to mix some alcohol with this, anything from a teaspoonful to a tablespoonful of brandy, but some homœopaths would say that is also unnecessary. Whichever way you do it, make sure you have screwed the lid on properly and then bash the bottle quite hard on a book or other hard surface 40 times. You then empty out the bottle completely, (keep all the mixture you empty out in one container; you should dispose of it carefully because it will be infectious with Bird flu for a few days). When emptying the bottle out completely I know many people want to make sure they can still see one drop of the mixture remaining in the bottom, but it does not have to be there as the residue on the sides of the inside of the bottle is more than enough to make the nosode. Refill the bottle with water (and alcohol if you want), hit it again 40 times. You continue the filling up, successing (hitting it 40 times) and emptying out a total of thirty times so you then end up with the nosode of Bird flu in approximately the 30th potency.

The Bird flu 30 nosode that you will have made is totally harmless and safe, just like any other homœopathic remedy, despite in its original undiluted state being a dangerous substance. It would be best for the final fill up to be done with only brandy, and then to transfer this to a new bottle with a dropper, which would be easier to use for medicating pilules. Some people are happy with the nosode being made in water with only a small amount of brandy as a preservative, but whenever I have made up other nosodes I have found they seem to be much more efficient and work better if they have been preserved totally in brandy, or mostly brandy, with only a small amount of water. This is your stock bottle and there should be plenty to last you and many others through the pandemic. You need four to five drops of this to medicate a 7gm or 8gm bottle of pilules; simply drop the drops into the bottle of pilules and give the bottle a little shake. It helps if the bottle is not quite full to the brim. Any more drops than that will be too much and the pilules will stick together and be difficult to get out of the bottle. You can buy unmedicated pilules from:

The Homœopathic Supply Company,
The Street, Bodham, Holt, Norfolk. NR25 6AD.
Tel: 01263 588788 email: orders@homeopathicsupply.com

Amongst other things, they also supply empty bottles of many different types and sizes, storage containers, and the book *Homœopathy: The Modern Prescriber* by Henrietta Wells.

Prevention and treatment using Bird flu Nosode 30

You can use the Bird flu nosode 30 for prevention and probably the simplest way is to take it twice a day for four days initially, then take one dose every fourth day for three more doses. After that take one dose twice a day on one day, every one to two weeks, or even just on one day a month, depending on how serious the disease has turned out to be, and how close it is to your area. Once the pandemic is over and if you have not had the disease, it might be a good idea to take a dose every two weeks throughout the winter in the same way that many people take other homœopathic flu prevention remedies. You could also take it at any time if there were reports of it in your area, or when travelling, if the disease were still a problem. If you are able to obtain the Bird flu nosode 30 for prevention, you will no longer need to take the Influenzinum, Pneumococcus, Bacillinum or Lueticum.

Additional remedies and advice for the acute treatment of Bird flu

You can also use Bird flu nosode 30 during the actual disease itself, whether it has been made by you or a homœopathic pharmacy, and this could be a great help to the patient. While you would be using the most similar remedy according to your symptoms as described elsewhere in this book, it would also be a good idea to take a dose of Bird flu nosode 30 twice a day for one to four days, if you get the illness. If you do this, you should leave at least half an hour, preferably an hour if you can, between the Bird flu 30 dose and any other homœopathic remedy you may be taking. You do not have to do this, but often using the appropriate nosode during an acute disease can assist enormously in getting better.

If Bird flu 30 is not available you could take the following additional remedies during Bird flu:

- In the initial stages take Influenzinum 30 twice a day for the first one to three days as this will help you throw it off.
- Should it develop into pneumonia then you should change from Influenzinum 30

to Pneumococcus 30 and take this twice a day, for a couple of days.
- If the pneumonia turns into the totally destructive phase of internal organs breaking down, then you should take Lueticum 30 twice a day for two days; you could always go back to taking Pneumococcus 30 again should it be necessary.

During each of the above scenarios you should not take the remedy concerned for more than two or three days, and it is unlikely to be required any longer. It should only be taken twice a day, and the dose should be taken first thing in the morning and last thing at night for whichever remedy you are on. You would then have the rest of the time free to take any of the homœopathic remedies that are indicated for your particular unique symptoms. You should not take more than one of the remedies above at any time because they each fit a different aspect of Bird flu. As said earlier, if a Bird flu nosode 30 has been made take this twice a day for up to four days instead of any of these remedies.

Genus Epidemicus

Many epidemics of acute diseases, not just of influenza, often have a particular remedy or group of remedies which seem to be more similar and therefore much more indicated than any others. So far the known symptoms of Bird flu appear to be most similar to Ant.Tart., Ipecac. and Sanguinaria. When the time comes and it is spread from human to human, there may be a greater emphasis on one of these; it is possible it could turn out to be other remedies, but nevertheless it is worth noting that, at the time of writing, these three remedies are the most indicated.

Comparing Bird flu with SARS

SARS can develop into pneumonia very fast and causes destruction of internal organs which is life threatening. This is very similar to the more serious symptoms of Bird flu. Both diseases have the usual flu symptoms at the beginning, a runny nose, sore throat, fever and chills, muscle aches and pains and probably a cough of some kind. However, with SARS there is less of the runny nose and sore throat with the flu symptoms, but everything else can be very like Bird flu. Both conditions can develop fever and cough symptoms, which can develop into pneumonia and the destruction of body tissue. It really does not matter which you happen to be treating with homœopathic treatment, because you are looking at the individual symptoms which are unique to the patient, and using these symptoms to choose the homœopathic remedies. The diagnosis in this case may only be useful in order to know what to expect in the way the disease progresses. This book could be just as useful for treating SARS as Bird flu. In SARS you would not use the remedy Influenzinum 30, nor would you use Bird flu nosode 30, but any of the other remedies could be indicated. You could of course make up a SARS nosode from the patient's sputum in a similar way to making the Bird flu Nosode.

Practical Preparations

As I said at the beginning of this book, in a Bird flu pandemic the outbreak is most likely to spread far and wide very quickly due to the frequency, extent and speed of travel these days. It is reasonable to assume that very quickly the hospitals will be overflowing with patients. If many people become ill, there could well be disruptions to many services. There could be some food shortages, petrol may become scarce, postal deliveries and rubbish collections may stop for a while; schools may close; public transport may become almost non-existent; there may even be power cuts and other shortages. By the time you realize this is happening it will already be too late to get prepared, so it would be best to start now. This sort of thing could happen with any pandemic, be it Bird flu, SARS or some other new disease.

The following is a list of a few basic things you should have in store (for the most extreme situations), but you will probably think of many other items that it would be sensible to add:

Protective mask, gloves, goggles and clothing (for when you go out). You can buy face masks and goggles and clothing from www.uksurvive.com and many other websites.

Rice – 1000gm is approximately one week's supply for one person, assuming that they are also able to obtain some meat to eat as well. 12 Kg will be sufficient for 12 weeks for one person.

Tins of meat – one half to two thirds of a 400 gm can of meat is enough for one person for one meal. Therefore you would need 45-60 tins approximately for one person for 12 weeks.

Mung beans, chick peas, lentils, sunflower sprouts, quinoa, pumpkin seeds, black eyed beans, aduki beans and alfalfa - all these dried foods store well, are very easy to grow, delicious and extremely nutritious. (If you are unfamiliar with how to use them there is a very helpful instruction book called *The Sprouters Handbook* by Edward Cairney, 2006.)

Tea bags – at least one a day per person.

Salt.

Loo rolls.

Tin opener.

Water containers such as new large plastic dustbins with lids and plastic jerry cans suitable for collecting water.

Matches and candles; torches and batteries.

Dog food.

Camping gas cooker with gas supplies, or calor gas supplies (although one hopes that it will never come to this, but there may well be power cuts).

Homœopathy: The Modern Prescriber by Henrietta Wells, 2002, so that you can treat any other acute condition that may crop up as well as Bird flu.

Any homœopathic remedies you think you might need from having read and studied that book.
Crataegus mother tincture and Calendula mother tincture (see below).
This book.
All the remedies mentioned on the Repertorization Chart in both a 30 and a 200. Buy them in 4gm bottles of pilules to get the best value for money.
In addition you should have the remedies mentioned in Chapter Six on Prevention, in 30s, and the remedies mentioned in Chapter Seven about after-effects of Bird Flu, in 30s.
You may want to have some of the remedies in the Repertorization Chart in 1Ms and 10Ms and very possibly some in 50Ms. Generally speaking get 1Ms if you are likely to be treating elderly not very energetic people and 10Ms if you are treating anyone energetic and younger; you could of course need both.

Water purification, wound cleaning and general cleanliness

Boiling water vigorously for five minutes is an excellent way of sterilizing it for drinking, but that may be impractical if there is a reduced supply of electricity or gas. Taking Crataegus mother tincture, five drops three times a day, does not cause side-effects and helps you resist any damaging bacteria. For children the dose would be less. You work it out by giving one fifth of the adult dose (one drop) per 10kg, or 22 lbs of the child's weight.

For cleaning wounds and injuries of all kinds you do not need to boil water if you use one teaspoonful of Calendula Mother Tincture per pint of water. For dressings dilute 25 parts water to one part Calendula Mother Tincture, and again you do not need to boil the water.

Keeping your hands meticulously clean is vitally important with many situations, but particularly with Bird flu. As mentioned earlier, it is very easy to get the conjunctivitis symptoms of Bird flu if you simply touch your eyes with your fingers.

Chapter Seven

Remedies for any after-effects of Bird flu

There are various things you can do to improve health for those who have had Bird flu. Probably the most important is to visit your homœopath and have some constitutional treatment to help your body to be strengthened after the weakening aspects of such an illness. However, there are a few remedies you should look at and choose the most similar one, depending on how you are and how the disease affected you. Gelsemium, Phos-ac., China and Kali Phos. are all remedies for extreme weakness and exhaustion following a severe illness.

Gelsemium This is a very useful remedy for the after-effects of any kind of flu and it is especially indicated for someone who is not only physically very weak but mentally apathetic. They can be trembling with weakness and nervousness, and find everything they try and do a great effort, although in fact most of the time they hardly do anything because they are so mentally dull and lacking in enthusiasm. Another indication for this remedy would be if the patient had needed it during their treatment for Bird flu itself at some stage. Gelsemium is also a good remedy for the after-effects of fright, fear and bad news; if those emotions applied to the patient during the course of the disease or afterwards, then this could be yet another reason for taking this remedy. You should also check out Gelsemium in the Materia Medica for a more detailed description.

Phos-ac. Again, like Gelsemium this remedy helps with weakness both physically and mentally. However, the cause of the weakness for Phos-ac. is usually a loss of bodily fluid. If during the course of having Bird flu the patient had lost a lot of fluid, either through having prolonged or profuse diarrhœa, profuse sweating, profuse urination or blood loss, then this remedy should be considered. It is also a remedy for the after-effects of shock and bad news like Gelsemium, but in Phos-ac. this also covers grief from losing someone you love. Here there may be utter despair. There is of course the possibility of this having happened during a Bird flu pandemic and so could be another reason for choosing Phos-ac. This remedy is also better for warmth and sleep, like Kali Phos., see below.

China Like Phos-ac., this remedy is useful when the weakness is due to loss of bodily fluids. It has all the extreme physical weakness of both Phos-ac. and Gelsemium, but it has far more digestive problems than these other two remedies. Certainly they have some digestive symptoms, but China has many more. It is a major liver remedy, can have a distended abdomen, much wind, bloating and colic and patients could be jaundiced. China is far more cross, irritable, oversensitive and sometimes just plain nasty, than just having the simple apathy of Gelsemium and Phos-ac. One of the reasons they can be so cross is that they feel they cannot think properly which makes them frustrated, and there is also much mental apathy.

Kali Phos. Like Gelsemium this remedy is indicated when the nervous system seems weakened, and both mentally and physically they are unable to do much, getting exhausted very quickly. The slightest mental effort seems to become a great task and something they find impossible to do. They tend to have spasms and twitches. Like Phos-ac., this remedy is better for warmth and sleep. Many discharges are very yellow, such as the urine, expectoration, skin (China) and stools. There could also be bloody stools. Sometimes if someone has needed Phos. during the acute disease, Kali Phos. may be one of the remedies indicated for the after-effects.

Tub.Aviaire This remedy is strongly indicated when the patient is left with an irritating dry cough after flu, particularly if the flu affected the lungs and had turned into bronchitis. It is particularly suited when the apices of the lungs are most affected, but if you are not sure whether this is the case, do not worry, because if it fits the symptoms in other ways it is still an excellent remedy. The cough is usually from a tickle, sounds dry, is fairly frequent and tires the person considerably. There is much debility generally and lack of appetite. There could still be slight fevers occurring, sweats and slightly bloody expectoration. Do not use lower than the 30th potency and the best dosage for it would be either (b) or (c) below. I find that, if following the (b) dosage, a ten to fourteen day break is best. If you use a 200, then one dose in the morning and evening and next morning, just three doses in total, is usually sufficient.

Dosage for after Bird flu remedies

There are many ways of prescribing for this type of situation and I describe some below. Choose which suits you best from the following.

a) Take the remedy in a 6 twice a day for seven to ten days. Repeat after a five day break if there is still a need for the remedy.

b) Take the remedy in a 30 twice a day for four days. Repeat after about a seven to ten day break, if there is still a need for the remedy.

c) Take the remedy in a 30 twice a day on one day a week for about a month.

Whichever of the above methods you choose, they are just a guide only. Remember that the remedy is simply taken to stimulate the body to heal itself, so that **as soon as there is improvement you should stop the remedy and only start again if there is a relapse** or if the patient is improved but not totally better, or may seem to have reached a plateau. Do not take two remedies at the same time if you think more than one is indicated, but *alternate* them. Remedies work much more efficiently if given separately. For instance you could prescribe China 6 twice a day for a week and then Phos-ac. 6 twice a day for a week. If prescribing Tub.Aviaire following (b) or (c) above, you could also prescribe any one of the other remedies, to be taken on the days off Tub.Aviare. If you do prescribe in this way with Tub.Aviaire, I find that taking the other remedy in a 6 is best.

Relationships for after-effects remedies

The following remedy relationships should be taken into consideration, although I do not think you will have much difficulty deciding which is most suitable. If in doubt you could always check with your homœopath.

China and Phos-ac. follow each other well and can be alternated.
Gelsemium can antidote China.
China can antidote Kali Phos.

Section Two

Homœopathic Bird Flu Repertory

This Homœopathic Repertory is a list of symptoms, or rubrics, which could occur in Bird flu. **The rubrics are taken mostly from the symptoms written in italics in the Materia Medica (in Section Three) as these are the key features for each remedy**. The way the Repertory is structured is by putting any detail of a rubric *following* its main heading, which is printed in bold. The remedies which have those symptoms in their remedy proving are listed in italics beside the rubric. The following details should help guide you:-

- Strong emotional symptoms come under Mentals, but delirium does not come under Mentals, it has its own separate heading.
- Parts of the body are usually under the named part, such as Back, Ears, Eyes, Face, Mouth etc.
- Symptoms concerning appearance of the face are under Face.
- Some throat symptoms come under Swallowing as well as Throat.
- Conjunctivitis and anything to do with vision or eyes, comes under Eyes.
- Symptoms about likes, dislikes, aggravations and ameliorations, concerning food or drink, are found under Digestion, appetite.
- Most symptoms concerning nausea, stools, etc., are entered under their own individual heading of Nausea, Stools, etc; occasionally they may be found under Digestion if relevant.
- Symptoms to do with the chest or the lungs come under Cough/Lungs, but pneumonia is under Pneumonia.
- Anything to do with the limbs comes under Extremities.
- Fevers and chills come under Fevers.
- There are numerous pain symptoms under the Pain heading, but any position or movement which makes any pain, or the patient generally, better or worse, comes under Position/Motion.

- Touch or pressure modalities affecting pain symptoms come under Touch and Pressure.
- Bleeding is under Discharges, bleeding.
- Symptoms concerning the time of day, night, early or late, age, speed of onset etc., are found under Time/Speed.
- Symptoms that affect a particular side, come under Side.
- The patient's reaction to any kind of temperature, weather or air, as well as his or her actual bodily temperature, will all be found under Weather, Body Temperature, Reactions to.

When using this Repertory, ***the only remedies included for each rubric are the ones which are indicated in flu or the known symptoms of Bird flu.*** In a full homœopathic repertory there are quite often literally hundreds of remedies for many of the rubrics ***so do not use this Repertory for anything other than flu or Bird flu.*** It does not give anything like enough remedies or rubric detail, and would be totally misleading if you tried using it for any other condition; you would end up making serious mistakes.

SYMPTOMS **REMEDIES**

Back:
chills in back and shivering: *Eup-perf.*
chills and heat run up and down: *Gels.*
heat comes up spine, heat between shoulder blades, coldness back of head: *Phos.*
pain, broken feeling, aching bones, worse motion: *Eup-perf.*
pain, lower back mainly, weak: *Kali-c.*
pain, lying on hard floor ameliorates: *Rhus-t.*
pain, muscular soreness, weakness: *Gels.*
pain, pressure ameliorates: *Rhus-t.*
pain, shoulder blade, inner angle right: *Chel.*
pain, stiff, lower back mainly; also body generally stiff: *Rhus-t.*
pain, violent, lower back: *Ant-t., Kali-c.* (see above).
pain, violent, heavy weight in coccyx area: *Ant-t.*
weakness: *Gels., Kali-c., Mur-ac.*
Breath: see also **Mouth.**
cold: *Camph., Carb-v.*
Causation:
abandoned, feeling of being: *Puls.*
alcohol/stimulants: *Lach., Nux-v.*
anger, effects of: *Ant-t., Bry.*
bad news: *Gels.*
bites and stings, allergic reaction to: *Apis, Carb-ac., Crot-h.*
cold, dry, windy weather, exposure to: *Acon., Hep-s.*
cold, extreme cold, exposure to: *Eup-perf.*
cold, wet weather, exposure to: *Bell., Nat-s., Rhus-t.*
cooling down suddenly when hot/sweaty: *Bell., Rhus-t.*
damp, hot or humid weather, mild winters: *Gels.*
damp living conditions: *Ant-t.*
drinking cold drinks in very hot weather: *Bry., Sulph.*
drinking dirty water: *Ars-a., Crot-h.*
drugs, bad effects from: *Ipec., Nit-ac., Nux-v.*
eating bad meat: *Ars-a., Carb-v., Pyrog.*
fear of disease: *Ars-a., Gels., Nit-ac.*
fear, fright or shock: *Acon., Bry., Camph., Crot-h., Gels., Verat-a.*
fluids, loss of: *Carb-v., (China, Phos-ac.).*
high altitudes, lack of oxygen: *Ars-a.*
hot sun, fright, lightning, alcohol, dirty water, sewage, vaccinations, insect stings: *Crot-h.*
hot weather, hot sun, exposure to: *Acon., Bell., Camph., Crot-h., Gels., Verat-a.*
injury: *Camph., Ferr-p., Nat-s.* (head), *Nit-ac.* (spine).

jealousy: *Lach., Puls.*
over-exertion and overheating: *Ars-a.*
sleep, loss of (e.g. from working at night), drugs and mercury: *Nit-ac., Nux-v.*
strains and overlifting: *Rhus-t.*
sun, exposure to too much: *Bell., Camph., Crot-h., Gels., Verat-v.*
suppressed catarrh: *Sang.*
suppressed discharge: *Bry., Ferr-p.* (sweat), *Lach., Puls., Sang., Sulph.*
suppressed eruption: *Apis, Bry., Ipec., Kali-c., Puls., Sulph., Verat-a.*
vaccinations: *Ant-t., Crot-h.*
wet feet, getting feet cold and wet: *Puls.*

Collapse: see also **Prostration**.
collapse: *Camph., Carb-v.*

Cough/Lungs:
air, air ameliorates cough and respiration: *Ars-a., Bapt., Carb-v., Puls.*
air, desire for, open window ameliorates: *Ars-a., Bapt., Carb-v., Puls.*
anger aggravates cough: *Ant-t.*
breathing difficult, faster than normal: *Phos.*
breathing difficult, panting: *Apis.*
breathing difficult, short of breath: *Acon., Ant-t., Apis, Ars-a., Bapt., Eup-perf., Gels.* (crowing), *Lach., Merc-s., Nit-ac., Nux-v., Phos., Puls., Sang.*
breathing difficult, worse for anything tight round throat: *Lach.*
breathing difficult, from pressure from stomach upwards, shallow and oppressed breathing: *Carb-v., Nux-v.*
burping ameliorates cough: *Sang.*
burping with cough, or with fullness in chest: *Verat-a.*
cold air aggravates: *Hep-s., Phos., Rhus-t.*
cold room aggravates: *Hep-s.*
coldness in chest: *Camph., Sulph.*
cough worse 4 am: *Ant-t.*
damp air ameliorates: *Acon., Hep-s.*
dry cough: *Acon., Apis, Ars-a., Bell., Bry., Crot-h., Ferr-p., Hep-s., Phos., Rhus-t.*
dry cough from dry throat, from tickle, worse at night: *Bell.*
dry cough in evening and night, loose in daytime: *Puls.*
dry cough with sore chest, spasm of larynx: *Gels.*
dry painful hacking cough: *Bry., Phos.*
dry teasing cough, worse during chill and worse putting hand out of bed: *Rhus-t.*
expectoration bloody or rusty: *Acon., Bry., Carb-v., Crot-h., Ferr-p., Ipec., Lach., Nit-ac., Phos., Rhus-t., Sang.*
expectoration bloody or rusty, which often tastes salty, sour, sweet or cold: *Phos.*
expectoration difficult and/or yellowy green: *Ars-i.*
expectoration difficult to raise: *Ant-t., Ars-i., Chel., Ipec., Kali-c., Sang.*
expectoration easy, bland, thick, yellow/cream/green mucus: *Puls.*

expectoration easy, much mucus in lungs, thick sticky yellow mucus: *Carb-v.*
expectoration frothy and scanty: *Ars-a.*
expectoration rusty: *Bry., Phos., Rhus-t., Sang.*
expectoration thick, ropy, greenish: *Nat-s.*
expectoration, smelly tough sputum: *Sang.*
gastric problems with cough: *Carb-v., Nux-v., Sang.*
headache brought on by cough: *Bry., Nux-v.*
later stages usually: *Ant-t.,* see also **Time/Speed**.
loose cough worse at night, cough with difficult breathing and sweat: *Eup-perf.*
loose cough, catarrhal mucus in chest: *Ant-t., Carb-v., Chel., Eup-perf., Hep-s., Ipec., Kali-c., Nat-s., Oscill., Puls., Sang., Sulph., Verat-a.*
loose in daytime, drier at night: *Puls.*
motion aggravates, worse deep inspiration: *Bry.*
night time aggravation, see also **Time/Speed**.
night time aggravation of tickle, dry cough from dry throat with tickle: *Bell.*
night time aggravation: *Acon., Eup-perf.*
night time aggravation, and after midnight, worse at 9 am or 9 pm: *Acon.*
pain in chest coming up from distended abdomen: *Carb-v., Nux-v.*
pain, burning heat in chest: *Phos.*
pain, burning heat in chest and circumscribed redness on chest, followed by diarrhœa: *Sang.*
pain, burning in chest, spasmodic cough: *Carb-v.*
pain, burning in chest, blue tinge to skin: *Carb-v.*
pain, burning or coldness in chest: *Ars-a., Sulph.*
pain, burning pain in chest from coughing: *Pyrog.*
pain, constricted feeling, needs to take a deep breath: *Lach.*
pain, constriction in chest, incessant, violent cough: *Ipec.*
pain, constriction of chest, tightness: *Bapt., Ipec., Lach., Phos.*
pain, darting, through upper third right lung: *Ars-a.*
pain, goes through left lung: *Nat-s.*
pain, sore chest with cough: *Eup-perf.*
pain, sore chest, spasm of throat: *Gels.*
pain, spasm of throat, dry cough with sore chest: *Gels.*
pain, spasmodic cough: *Sang.*
pain, stabbing stitching pains in lungs: *Ars-a.* (darts), *Bry., Kali-c.*
pain, stabbing stitching pains independent of respiration (*Bry.* pain is worse for respiration): *Kali-c.*
pain, stabbing stitching pains on left side: *Phos.*
pain, weight on chest, pressure, oppression: *Lach., Phos., Puls., Sulph.*
pain, plug/lump sensation, moves up and down throat with the cough: *Lach.*
position, has to sit up to cough: *Ant-t., Ars-a., Bry., Hep-s., Puls., Pyrog.*
position, holds chest when coughing: *Bry., Eup-perf., Nat-s.*

position, lies with head back: *Ant-t., Hep-s.*
position, lying down aggravates cough: *Ant-t., Ars-a., Bry., Hep-s., Puls., Pyrog.*
position, lying left side aggravates cough: *Eup-perf., Phos.*
position, lying on left side aggravates breathing but lying on right side aggravates cough: *Merc-s.*
rattling in chest, loose cough: *Ant-t., Chel., Carb-v., Hep-s., Ipec., Kali-c., Nat-s., Puls.* (dry at night), *Sang., Sulph., Verat-a.*
rattling of much mucus in chest which cannot raise: *Ant-t., Ipec., Kali-c., Sang.*
stuffy room aggravates: *Puls.*
suffocating feeling: *Ant-t., Bapt., Lach.*
trembles with cough: *Phos.*
uncovering aggravates: *Hep-s., Rhus-t.*
voice, high: *Bell.*
voice, hoarse: *Acon., Bell., Carb-v., Eup-perf., Hep-s., Ipec., Phos., Rhus-t.*
voice hoarse and croupy: *Acon., Hep-s.*
voice hoarse, worse evening: *Carb-v., Phos., Rhus-t.*
warm room aggravates: *Bry., Puls., Pyrog., Verat-a.*
warm room aggravates when entering from cold, and cold when entering from warm: *Phos.*

Delirium: see also **Mentals.**
Acon., Ant-t., Apis, Ars-a., Bapt., Bell., Bry., Camph., Carb-ac., Carb-v., Chel., Crot-h., Gels., Hep-s., Ipec., Kali-c., Lach., Merc-s., Mur-ac., Nit-ac., Nux-v., Phos., Puls., Rhus-t., Sulph., Verat-a., Verat-v.

Digestion: see also **Stools**.
appetite, aggravated by milk: *Nit-ac., Oscill., Sulph.*
appetite, aggravated by rich food, worse wine, averse fats, fullness feeling: *Carb-v.*
appetite, aggravated by rich foods: *Carb-v., Puls.*
appetite, aggravated by salt, having too much salt: *Phos.*
appetite, aggravated by warm food: *Puls.*
appetite, ameliorated by warm drinks: *Nux-v.*
appetite, averse to meat and sweet things: *Nit-ac.*
appetite, desires apples, fruits, acids: *Ant-t.*
appetite, desires cold drinks and cold snacks: *Camph., Merc-s.* (drinks).
appetite, desires fats/stimulants: *Nux-v.*
appetite, desires indigestible things, chalk, earth: *Nit-ac.*
appetite, desires milk: *Apis, Rhus-t.*
appetite, desires rich food, pastry and cream although they aggravate: *Puls.*
appetite, desires salt. Worse too much salt: *Phos.*
appetite, desires stimulants: *Carb-ac., Nux-v.*
appetite, desires warm food and drink only: *Chel.*
cough, eating or drinking aggravate cough: *Bry.*
diarrhœa: see **Stools**.

distension in abdomen, contraction in, and pain extends to chest: *Carb-v., Nux-v.*
distension, bloating several hours after food: *Nux-v.*
distension, very windy, colic, fullness: *Carb-v.*
hiccoughs: *Eup-perf., Nux-v., Verat-v.*
liver problems: *Ars-a., Chel., Crot-h., Nux-v.*
nausea, no better vomiting, constant nausea: *Ipec.*
nausea, on sight or smell of food: *Ars-a., Eup-perf.*
nausea, on slightest movement: *Bry.*
nausea, retching and vomiting, nausea in waves: *Ant-t.*
nausea, stomach as if full of water, sour belching: *Kali-c.*
pain abdomen, right side, is sensitive and painful with rumbling: *Bapt.*
pain around navel: *Ipec.*
pain: see also **Touch and pressure**
pain spasms: *Verat-v.*
pain stomach, empty, gone, weak sensation: *Phos.*
pain stomach, as of a stone: *Bry., Nux-v.*
pain stomach, heavy feeling: *Puls.*
pain stomach/abdomen burning: *Ars-a., Carb-ac.*
pain stomach/abdomen, as of a weight, worse eating: *Nux-v.*
pain stomach/abdomen wind and hiccoughs: *Nux-v.*
pain stomach/abdomen, bruised soreness of abdominal walls, sore bowels, wind, distension: *Nux-v.*
pain stomach/abdomen, cold, icy cold feeling: *Verat-a.*
pain stomach/abdomen, colicky: *Acon., Carb-v.*
pain stomach/abdomen, contractions in distended abdomen, pain extends to chest: *Carb-v., Nux-v.*
pain stomach/abdomen, cramping: *Ars-a.*
pain stomach/abdomen, pressure of clothes aggravate: *Crot-h., Lach.*
pain stomach/abdomen, sinking feeling in stomach, pain right side abdomen, rumbles: *Bapt.*
pain stomach/abdomen, slight touch aggravates, better for hard pressure: *Bry.*
slow digestion: *Carb-v.*
stomach as if full of water, sour belching: *Kali-c.*
taste, bitter taste: *Bry., Puls., Sulph.*
taste, metallic: *Merc-s.*
taste, sweet: *Merc-s., Puls.*
thirst: *Acon., Ars-a.* (sips only), *Bell., Bry., Eup-perf., Ferr-p., Merc-s., Nux-v., Phos., Rhus-t., Verat-a.*
thirst, chill, during, thirstless during fever: *Nux-v.*
thirst despite profuse saliva: *Merc-s.*
thirst for cold drinks and cold snacks: *Camph.*

thirst for cold drinks but vomits as soon as it warms in the stomach (also may vomit cold food): *Ars-a., Phos., Verat-a.*
thirst for cold drinks, prefers beer, worse for milk: *Acon.*
thirst for cold drinks, thirst for beer, continuous hunger: *Merc-s.*
thirst for cold water, followed by shuddering and vomiting of bile, food and drink: *Eup-perf.*
thirst, very thirsty for cold: *Acon., Ars-a., Bry., Camph., Eup-perf., Ferr-p., Lach.* (mainly because ameliorates the throat pain), *Merc-s., Phos.*
thirst for large quantities at a time, usually of water: *Bry.*
thirst for lemonade or water particularly: *Bell.*
thirst for sips of water only: *Ant-t., Ars-a.*
thirst, extremely thirsty: *Bell., Bry., Ferr-p., Phos., Rhus-t.*
thirst, hot drinks which ameliorate nausea: *Nux-v.*
thirst, warm drink and food only: *Chel.*
thirstless usually: *Ant-t., Apis., Gels., Ipec., Puls.*
thirstless, but may be thirsty during sweat: *Gels.*
thirstless, dry mouth, despite having dry mouth: *Gels., Puls.*
thirstless, high fever, during: *Bell., Gels., Ipec., Nux-v.*
vomiting and diarrhœa at the same time, or almost at the same time: *Ars-a.*
vomiting copious and violent: *Verat-a.*
vomiting immediately after drinking, particularly after drinking cold water: *Ars-a., Phos., Verat-a.*
vomiting of bile, food and drink; after drinking cold water; thirst for cold water: *Eup-perf.*
vomiting of black or coffee ground type vomit or of blood: *Crot-h.*
vomiting undigested food. Sour burping: *Ferr-p.*
vomiting with fear, profuse sweat and increased urination: *Acon.*
vomiting with nausea and much retching: *Ant-t., Nux-v.*

Discharges: see **Stools,** and also see **Sweats.**
acrid and burning: *Ars-a., Ars-i., Carb-v., Carb-ac., Merc-s., Nit-ac., Nux-v., Sulph.*
acrid and corrosive from rectum: *Carb-v.*
acrid from eyes: *Ars-a., Ars-i., Merc-s., Sulph.*
acrid, bloody: *Nux-v., Sulph.*
acrid, thick: *Ars-i., Merc-s., Nit-ac.*
acrid, thick, yellow and smelly: *Nit-ac.*
acrid, thin and smelly: *Nit-ac.*
acrid, thin usually, excoriating and burning making skin sore: *Ars-a., Ars-i., Nit-ac., Sulph.*
acrid, usually, green and smelly (particularly from nose), yellow and smelly (particularly from ears): *Merc-s.*
better for discharges always: *Lach., Nux-v.*

better for passing wind and burping: *Sang.*
better for profuse urination in headache: *Gels.*
bland, thick discharges, green, yellow, cream, white: *Arg-n., Hep-s., Puls.*
bland, thick, green, yellow, white, cream, but changeable: *Puls.*
bleeding bright red blood: *Ferr-p., Ipec., Nit-ac., Phos.*
bleeding through skin, bloody sweat: *Crot-h.*
bleeding: *Carb-v., Crot-h., Ferr-p., Ipec., Lach., Mur-ac., Nit-ac., Phos., Sulph.*
bleeding, black blood, stringy blood, oozing blood: *Crot-h.*
bleeding, bright red blood or like bloody water: *Nit-ac.*
bleeding, bright ref profuse haemorrhages, gushing: *Ipec.*
bleeding, dark oozing blood: *Carb-v., Crot-h.*
bleeding, from anywhere: *Crot-h., Phos.*
bleeding, like coffee grounds (also stools): *Crot-h.*
bleeding, thin blood containing particles like straw: *Lach.*
copious, stools, urine, vomit, saliva, sweat: *Verat-a.*
smelly and putrid: *Ars-a., Bapt., Carb-ac., Carb-v., Crot-h., Hep-s., Merc-s., Nit-ac., Pyrog., Sulph.*
sweats, better when sweats come as fever breaks; otherwise very dry throughout: *Acon.*
yellow from eyes: *Oscill.*

Dryness: running through remedy: *Acon., Bry.*

Early: see also **Time/Speed**.
early stages: *Acon., Bell., Camph., Ferr-p., Oscill.*

Ears:
blood oozes from: *Crot-h.*
inflammation of, early stages: *Acon., Bell., Ferr-p.*
pain sharp and scratchy and cutting: *Hep-s.*
thick, yellow smelly discharge: *Hep-s., Merc-s.*
thick, yellow, creamy discharge: *Puls.*

Exhaustion: see also **Prostration**.
extreme: *Ant-t., Ars-a., Bapt., Camph., Carb-v., Gels., Kali-c., Verat-a.*

Extremities:
extremities, cold: *Acon.* (feet), *Ars-a., Bell., Camph., Carb-v.*
cold from knees downwards: *Carb-v.*
hot and sweaty hands and feet: *Sulph.*
hot hands and cold feet: *Acon.*
joints red and swollen: *Bry.*
joints may give way suddenly, arms and hands go numb easily: *Phos.*
pain, aching limbs: *Nux-v.*
pain, aching soreness as if bones broken: *Eup-perf.*
pain, burning palms and/or soles: *Sang., Sulph.*
pain, limb pains move around, worse letting affected part hang down: *Puls.*

pain, limbs heavy and aching muscles and soreness, bed feels too hard, part lain on feels sore and bruised: *Bapt., Pyrog.*
pain, limbs, jerks and spasms, cold: *Bell.*
pain, numb and tingling: *Acon.*
pain, right shoulder: *Sang.*
pain, soles very sensitive if touched: *Kali-c.*
pain, stiffness, tearing and aching of muscles and joints and bones, restless: *Rhus-t.*
pain, stitching and tearing pains anywhere: *Bry.*
red patch below little finger on palm: *Acon.*
restless and cold: *Ars-a.*
weak and exhausted muscles: *Kali-c., Mur-ac.*
weak and trembling, muscular soreness: *Gels.*
weak and trembling, particularly hands: *Merc-s.*

Eyes:
bleeding from, helps re-absorption: *Crot-h.*
bloodshot: *Apis, Arg-n., Crot-h., Ferr-p., Merc-s., Sulph.*
conjunctivitis with acrid discharge: *Ars-a., Merc-s., Sulph.*
conjunctivitis, red and inflamed eyes: *Arg-n., Ipec., Merc-s., Puls., Sulph.*
conjunctivitis, thick pustular discharge: *Arg-n., Hep-s., Puls.*
conjunctivitis, yellow discharges mostly during early stage of flu: *Oscill.*
contracted pupils: *Acon.*
dilated pupils: *Bell., Verat-v.*
eyelids puffy: *Apis.*
heavy with drooping lids: *Bapt., Gels.*
inflammation of eyes, and around eyes: *Rhus-t.*
letters appear red: *Phos.*
pain, aches, twitching of eyes: *Gels.*
pain, burning acrid discharge: *Ars-a., Ars-i., Merc-s.*
pain, eyeballs sore: *Eup-perf.*
pain, from headache travels to right eye: *Sang.*
pain, neuralgia of eyes and of the bones round eyes: *Crot-h., Merc-s.*
pain, sharp stitching pains: *Apis, Camph., Nit-ac.*
pain, weep and run with the pains: *Apis, Ipec., Nit-ac.*
photophobia: *Acon., Apis, Ars-a., Bapt., Bell., Crot-h., Nit-ac., Nux-v., Phos., Sang.*
photophobia, with burning eyes or with hot acrid tears: *Ars-a.*
pustular inflammations of eye: *Rhus-t.*
tears hot: *Apis, Ars-a.*
vision blurred and/or dizzy: *Gels.*
watering, swollen lids, red: *Acon., Apis.*
weep and watering: *Acon., Ars-a., Nit-ac.*

Face: conjunctivitis, see **Eyes.**

discolouration, alternates between being flushed and pale: *Ferr-p.*

discolouration blue, cold, covered with cold sweat, incessant quivering chin or lower jaw, blue/black/grey look around mouth, lips, nostrils and maybe eyes too: *Ant-t.*

discolouration, blue: *Ant-t., Camph., Carb-v., Verat-a.*

discolouration, blue colour, persistent nosebleed, breath cold, tongue cold: *Camph.*

discolouration, bluey red or purple, swollen and puffed: *Bapt., Lach.*

discolouration, circumscribed redness of cheeks: *Sang., Sulph.*

discolouration, circumscribed redness of cheeks; hectic flush of cheeks with burning: *Sang.*

discolouration, dark red: *Bapt.* (dusky, besotted look), *Mur-ac.*

discolouration, hot and flushed with heavy stupefied look, droopy eyelids: *Gels.*

discolouration, may be fiery red, shiny: *Bell.*

discolouration, one cheek red, one pale: *Acon.*

discolouration, pale blue/grey round eyes and lips: *Ipec.*

discolouration, pale on sitting up: *Acon., Verat-v.*

discolouration, pale or blue: *Carb-v., Verat-a.*

discolouration, pale round nose and mouth: *Carb-ac.*

discolouration, pale yellow: *Ars-a.*

discolouration, pale, earthy; dribbling: *Merc-s.*

discolouration, red: *Bell., Bry., Verat-v.*

discolouration, very red lips, circumscribed redness of cheeks: *Sulph.*

discolouration, yellow, sickly: *Nit-ac.*

discolouration, yellow jaundiced: *Chel.*

lips, corners of mouth cracked and scabby, peeling lips: *Nit-ac.*

lips, cracked and scabby: *Bapt., Carb-v., Mur-ac.*

lips, dry cracked bleeding, ulcerated lips: *Bapt.*

lips, dry, peeling, cracked: *Bry., Carb-v., Nit-ac.*

lips, fever blisters and cold sores: *Rhus-t.*

old-looking: *Ars-a.*

pains needle-like burning pains: *Ars-a.*

swellings, puffy, like a bag of water: *Apis.*

swollen, jaws crack when chewing, nosebleeds, inflamed eyes, tongue coated with triangular clear red tip/diagonally red: *Rhus-t.*

Fever:

chill alternating with heat: *Ipec.*

chill alternating with heat, icy coldness with burning in various parts too. Icy cold or hot sweat: *Carb-v.*

chill alternating with heat, rapid changes in temperature: *Verat-a., Verat-v.*

chill and heat chase each other up and down back: *Gels.*

chill cold and icy with burning in various parts: *Carb-v.*
chill continuously: *Nit-ac.*
chill externally, and internally hot and burning: *Ars-a.*
chill from slightest draught: *Hep-s., Rhus-t.*
chill in back and shivering: *Eup-perf., Gels.*
chill or fever, cold with hot head and red face: *Bry.*
chill or heat, wants to be held as shakes so much: *Gels.*
chill, uncovering, desire for (except during heat): *Camph.*
chill with thirst, fever with thirstlessness: *Nux-v.*
chill worse at 4 pm, worse for heat and worse if moves: *Apis.*
chill worse at 4 pm. External heat aggravates, desires fresh air: *Puls.*
chill worse in warm room: *Ipec., Puls.*
clammy profuse sweat all over: *Ant-t.*
cold, freezing inside despite fever, must be covered up: *Bell., Nux-v.*
cold, icy cold in patches: *Ars-a.*
cold, icy coldness of whole body: *Camph.*
cold, icy water or hot burning water running through veins, as if: *Ars-a.*
early stages: see also **Time/Speed**.
early stages: *Acon., Bell., Ferr-p.*
flushes of heat frequently, dry skin and thirst, sweat in single parts or one side of body: *Sulph.*
gastric: *Acon., Ant-t., Ars-a., Bapt., Bell., Bry., Carb-v., Chel., Eup-perf., Gels., Ipec., Merc-s., Mur-ac., Nat-s., Nux-v., Phos., Puls., Rhus-t., Sulph., Verat-a.*
heat aggravates, desires fresh air: *Puls.*
heat and burning swelling redness, shiny, dry (before sweat): *Bell.*
heat without thirst: *Ipec.*
heat, better uncovering: *Acon., Mur-ac.*
heat, dry and burning: *Bry.*
heat, freezing inside: *Bell., Nux-v.*
heat: see also **Weather, Body Temperature, Reactions to.**
heat, very hot but may have no thirst during fever: *Bell.*
heat, very hot with hot head and cold limbs: *Bell.*
heat, very hot with waves of coldness: *Acon., Ars-a.*
heat, waves of heat through body: *Sulph.*
heat, worse if heated: *Merc-s., Puls.*
heat, worse uncovering (hot stage): *Bell., Camph., Hep-s., Nux-v., Rhus-t.*
pains, in bones precede the chill and thirst: *Eup-perf.*
pains, muscular soreness: *Eup-perf.* (but mostly bones), *Gels., Rhus-t.*
pains, restless, stiff and sore with fever, worse uncovering; desire to stretch; chilly: *Rhus-t.*
septic fevers: *Ant-t., Apis., Ars-a., Bapt., Bry., Carb-v., Carb-ac., Crot-h., Lach., Merc-s., Mur-ac., Phos., Puls., Pyrog., Rhus-t., Sulph.*

sudden onset of fever: *Acon., Bapt., Bell., Ferr-p.*
shakes so much needs to be held: *Gels.*
sweats: see also **Sweats.**
sweats profusely but without relief: *Merc-s., Pyrog., Sulph.*
sweats profusely when fever breaks: *Bry.*
sweats, bloody: *Crot-h.*
sweats, drenching at night: *Ars-i.*
thirst in fever: see also **Digestion**, thirst.
thirstless during fever: *Bell.* (sometimes), *Gels., Ipec., Nux-v.*
thirstless during fever and chill: *Puls.*
thirstless during fever, but chill with thirst: *Nux-v.*
trembling: *Camph.* (with cold), *Gels.* (needs to be held).
uncovering aggravates: *Bell., Camph.* (hot stage), *Hep-s., Nux-v., Rhus-t.*
uncovering aggravates, cold inside despite fever: *Bell., Nux-v., Rhus-t.*
uncovering ameliorates, during heat: *Acon., Mur-ac.*
uncovering desire for, during chill, (not during heat): *Camph.*

Glands:
swollen, red shiny hot and dry: *Bell.*

Head:
occiput (back of head), coldness of: *Phos.*
scalp sore and hair falls out easily: *Carb-v.*

Headache:
pain, as if bandaged, tension on scalp: *Merc-s.*
pain, band, like a band round head: *Gels., Nit-ac.*
pain, better for pressure and worse any movement, holds head, must lie down: *Bry.*
pain, better sitting half propped or worse lying flat: *Bell., Eup-perf., Gels.*
pain, brain feels loose, striking against skull: *Rhus-t.*
pain, bursting from neck up over head to eyes/forehead: *Gels.*
pain, from coughing: *Bry., Nux-v.*
pain, in temple extending to ear: *Gels.*
pain, numb, feels heavy, numb and large: *Bapt.*
pain, occiput (back of head): *Camph., Eup-perf., Gels., Phos., Rhus-t., Sang., Verat-v.*
pain, presses head into pillow: *Sang., Apis.*
pain, pressing, feels as if eyes would be pressed out: *Sang.*
pain, pressure on top of head, or burning: *Sulph.*
pain, pulsating hot and bursting: *Acon.*
pain, pulsating occiput synchronious with pulse: *Camph.*
pain, pulsating throbbing: *Acon., Bell., Camph., Sang., Verat-v.*
pain, rolls head from side to side with pain: *Apis.*
pain, stabbing, stinging: *Apis.*

pain, stitching, cutting pains: *Bry., Camph.*
pain, stitching in temples and around eyes: *Camph.*
pain, top of head: *Lach., Sulph.*
pain, top of head icy cold and on face: *Verat-a.*
pains, sharp and throbbing, rush of blood to head with nausea and faintness: *Sang.*
periodicity every 7th day: *Sang.*
photophobia with headache: *Sang.*
sick headache, ascends from occiput (back of head) area to over the right eye: *Sang.*
sick headache, bilious, with nausea, pain at back of head from lying down with sense of weight in occiput (back of head): *Eup-perf.*
starts in morning increases to noon then diminishes: *Sang.*

Heart:
beat felt through body: *Pyrog., Verat-v.*
failure in septic states: *Pyrog.*
feels must keep moving or heart will stop: *Gels.*
palpitations and trembling when still: *Rhus-t.*
palpitations with anxiety: *Acon., Phos.*
palpitations with anxiety with pains in left shoulder: *Acon.*
palpitations, fast or slow pulse, out of proportion to fever: *Pyrog.*

Light:
aggravates: *Acon., Ars-a., Bapt., Bell., Crot-h., Nit-ac., Nux-v., Phos., Sang.*

Margins:
affects margins of any outlet, i.e. of mouth, eyes, throat, anus: *Nit-ac.*

Mentals: see also **Delirium.**
alone aggravates, better company: *Ars-a., Camph., Nux-v., Phos., Puls.*
anger aggravates the cough: *Ant-t.*
angry and irritable: *Bell., Nit-ac., Sang.*
anxiety: *Acon., Ars-a., Bry.* (about business), *Camph.*
apathy: *Gels.*
changeable moods, from tears to laughter and back again: *Puls.*
confusion: see also **Delirium**.
confusion: *Bapt., Bry., Crot-h., Lach., Sang.*
confusion, wants to go home when at home: *Bry.*
constantly changing their mind: *Merc-s., Puls.*
cross, impatient and irritable, worse alone, zealous, fiery mood: *Nux-v.*
crying out: *Apis.*
desires company, excitable, impressionable, sympathetic and loves sympathy: *Phos.*
fastidious: *Apis., Ars-a., Nux-v.*
fear of dark: *Phos.*

fears death: *Acon., Ars-a., Nit-ac.*
fears disease: *Ars-a., Gels., Nit-ac.*
fears going to sleep, always worse after sleep: *Lach.*
fears, anticipatory fears, e.g. of the disease, shaking, trembling with fear, or apathetic: *Gels.*
fears, easily frightened and startled: *Carb-v.*
fears, full of fears and over-active imagination, fear of ghosts: *Kali-c.*
fears, intense fear: *Acon., Ars-a., Kali-c., Phos.*
fears, poison, apprehension worse at night, cannot remain in bed: *Rhus-t.*
hypersensitive to light, noise, and all impressions: *Bell.*
imagines himself a great person, self-centred and selfish: *Sulph.*
impatient: *Hep-s., Nux-v.*
indecision, poor self confidence: *Merc-s., Puls.*
indifference, dwell on imaginary misfortune: *Verat-a.*
irritable or apathetic: *Ant-t.*
irritable, touchy: *Ant-t., Bell., Bry., Hep-s., Nit-ac., Nux-v.*
jealous: *Apis, Lach., Puls.*
loquacity, suspicion: *Lach., Verat-v.*
manipulative: *Puls.*
mild, gentle, tearful, weepy, desires sympathy/attention: *Puls.*
moaning or silent: *Mur-ac.*
restlessness: *Acon., Apis, Ars-a., Bapt., Bell., Mur-ac., Pyrog., Rhus-t., Sulph.*
sad and low: *Nat-s.*
sluggish and slow: *Apis, Carb-v.*
sympathy, desire for: *Phos., Puls.*
thinks he is broken or double and tosses around in bed to gather the pieces together, confusion; restlessness or stupor; falls asleep while speaking; as if drunk; delirium: *Bapt.*
vexation, reserved displeasure: *Ipec.*
weeping: *Apis, Crot-h., Puls.*

Mouth:
bleeding from: *Crot-h., Ipec.*
breath cold: *Camph., Carb-v.*
breath odour, putrid smelly breath, dry parched brown centre of tongue, cracked and ulcerated: *Bapt.*
breath smelly: *Ars-a., Bapt., Carb-v., Carb-ac., Chel., Crot-h., Lach., Merc-s., Mur-ac., Nux-v., Pyrog.*
burning from mouth to stomach: *Carb-ac.*
chewing motion of jaws: *Bell., Bry.*
dry: *Acon., Bapt., Bry., Gels., Puls., Pyrog.*
dry and parched: *Bapt., Bry.*
dry but no thirst: *Gels., Puls.*

gums, bleeding gums: *Ant-t., Ars-a., Carb-v., Crot-h., Hep-s., Lach., Merc-s., Mur-ac., Nit-ac., Nux-v., Phos., Sulph.*
gums, bleeding, taste bitter, saliva bloody: *Nux-v., Sulph.*
saliva increased: *Crot-h., Merc-s.*
saliva increased, but still thirsty: *Merc-s.*
sordes on teeth and lips. Ulcers: *Mur-ac.*
taste, bitter: *Bry., Nux-v., Puls., Sulph.*
taste, metallic: *Merc-s.*
taste, sweet: *Puls., Merc-s.*
tongue, brown streak down centre: *Bapt., Pyrog.*
tongue, burning pain with brown centre: *Bapt.*
tongue, cleanish tongue despite the vomiting and digestive problems: *Ipec.*
tongue, coated with very red clear triangular tip or diagonally red: *Rhus-t.*
tongue, cold: *Camph.*
tongue, dry tongue and throat, dry parched cracked lips: *Bry.*
tongue, indented by teeth, furrowed lengthwise, yellow and flabby, ulcers: *Merc-s.*
tongue, shiny dry large flabby and red and clean and smooth, brown streak down centre of tongue: *Pyrog.*
tongue, stiff, difficult to talk: *Crot-h.*
tongue, strawberry-like: *Bell.*
tongue, tastes bitter, brown coating on: *Nat-s.*
tongue, thick white coating, may have red edges or streaks: *Ant-t.*
tongue, yellow/white mucus on: *Puls.*
ulcers and denuded spots, bluish purplish gums and easy bleeding: *Lach.*
ulcers with splinter-like pains: *Nit-ac.*
ulcers: *Ars-a., Bapt., Lach., Merc-s., Mur-ac., Nit-ac.*

Nausea: *Ant-t., Ars-a., Bapt., Bry., Eup-perf., Ipec., Kali-c., Nux-v., Sang.*
faintness with nausea worse motion: *Bry.*
hot drinks ameliorate nausea: *Nux-v.*
persistent nausea with vomiting, but no better for vomiting: *Ipec.*
sight, smell, thought of food cause nausea: *Ars-a., Eup-perf., Ipec.*
smell of flowers cause nausea: *Sang.*
vomiting ameliorates nausea: *Ant-t.*
vomiting with much retching and nausea: *Nux-v.*

Noise:
aggravates: *Acon., Bell., Nit-ac., Nux-v.*

Nose:
bleeding: *Acon., Ant-t., Bell., Bry., Camph., Carb-v., Crot-h., Ferr-p., Hep-s., Ipec., Kali-c., Lach., Merc-s.* (from violence of cough), *Mur-ac., Nat-s., Nit-ac., Nux-v., Phos., Puls., Pyrog., Rhus-t., Sulph., Verat-a.*
bleeding daily, with pale face: *Carb-v.*
bleeding, black blood and stringy blood: *Crot-h.*

bleeding, persistent: *Camph.*
bleeding, with cough: *Ipec., Merc-s.*
bleeding, dark, clotted blood with chest problems: *Nit-ac.*
discharge, acrid catarrhal, burning: *Ars-i.*
discharge, greenish, smelly: *Merc-s.*
discharge, smelly, yellow, catarrhal corrosive: *Nit-ac.*
discharge, thick and yellow with salty mucus: *Nat-s.*
discharge, thick yellow, cream, green, bland: *Puls.*
discharge, watery: *Acon.*
dry and sensitive to smell: *Acon.*
dry catarrh, scabby and easy bleeding: *Sulph.*
raw, ulcerated, swelling and decay of nasal bones: *Merc-s.*
red and swollen at tip: *Apis.*
sensitive to smell, extremely: *Carb-ac.*
stuffed up at night and out of doors: *Nux-v.*
stuffed up in warm room, ulcerated nostrils: *Kali-c.*
ulcerated nostils: *Ant-t., Merc-s., Kali-c.*

Pain:
aching, and soreness: *Eup-perf., Gels., Rhus-t.*
aching, weakness and tremors: *Gels.*
as if bandaged (head): *Merc-s.*
band (round head): *Gels., Nit-ac.*
bed feels too hard: *Bapt.*
better passing wind, better for burping: *Sang.*
broken, as if back were broken, worse motion, aching, sore: *Eup-perf.*
bruised, sore, aching, weak although restless: *Pyrog.*
burning: *Acon., Ars-a., Ars-i., Carb-ac., Carb-v.* (in chest with cough), *Mur-ac., Phos., Pyrog.* (in throat and lungs from cough), *Sang., Sulph., Verat-v.*
burning, as if hot water poured over part: *Sang.*
burning, better for heat: *Ars-a.*
burning, in chest although otherwise cold: *Carb-v.*
burning, itching, weight on chest: *Sulph.*
burning, pulsations, congestion of blood to head, chest and abdomen: *Sang.*
burning, stinging and prickling: *Apis.*
burning, stomach with gastric problems: *Sang.*
bursting: *Bry.*
changeable, modalities change, and changes place frequently: *Puls.*
constriction: *Lach.*
cramp: *Ars-a., Bell., Camph., Oscill., Verat-a.*
heat and burning running through remedy: *Acon.*
heaviness, aching and soreness: *Eup-perf., Gels.*
hypersensitive to: *Kali-c.*

itching: *Carb-ac., Sulph.*
movement aggravates: *Bry.*
numbness: *Acon.*
painlessness: *Carb-ac.*
pressing: *Lach.*
rawness: *Ars-a., Merc-s., Sulph.*
restlessness with pain: *Ars-a., Pyrog., Rhus-t.*
restlessness, worse initial motion, better continued motion, worse over-exertion: *Rhus-t.*
round navel: *Ipec.*
sharp throbbing pains in headache: *Sang.*
sensation as of a lump in the part: *Lach.*
sick feeling all over: *Bapt.*
soreness, stiffness and aching of muscles more than bones, restless with the pain, cannot get comfortable: *Rhus-t.*
soreness causing restlessness then exhaustion: *Mur-ac.*
soreness internally and extreme aching of bones with sore flesh: *Eup-perf.*
soreness, rawness, burning, itching: *Sulph.*
soreness, tearing and extreme aching particularly of eyes and bones: *Eup-perf.*
spasms and oversensitiveness: *Bell., Nux-v.*
sticking, splinter-like pains: *Arg-n., Hep-s., Nit-ac.*
stiffness of muscles and back: *Rhus-t.*
stinging, prickling and burning: *Apis.*
stitching, tearing, cutting, stabbing: *Bry., Chel., Kali-c.*
stool, urging to pass stool with every pain: *Nux-v.*
tearing: *Eup-perf., Rhus-t.*
throbbing: *Bell., Sulph., Verat-v.*
throbbing pulsating, sharp, cutting or shooting: *Bell.*
tingling: *Acon.*
weight, pressure, oppression, tight: *Phos.*

Painlessness: *Bapt.* (inflamed throat), *Carb-ac.*

Pneumonia: *Acon., Ant-t., Ars-a., Ars-i., Bry., Carb-v., Chel., Ferr-p., Hep-s., Ipec., Kali-c., Lach., Merc-s., Nat-s., Phos., Puls., Pyrog., Rhus-t., Sang., Sulph., Verat-v.*
left lung: *Acon., Lach., Nat-s., Phos., Sang.* (but usually worse on right side).
lower left lung: *Nat-s., Phos.*
lower right lung: *Kali-c., Merc-s.*
right lung: *Ars-a., Bell., Bry., Chel., Kali-c., Merc-s., Phos., Sang., Sulph.*
upper left lung: *Acon.*
upper right lung: *Ars-a., Chel.*
when not clearing up: *Ars-i.*
with jaundice: *Merc-s.*

Position/Motion:

cough and hoarseness, better for getting onto hands and knees, on all fours: *Eup-perf.*

cough, sits up to cough: *Ant-t., Ars-a., Bry., Puls., Pyrog.*

jarring aggravates: *Bell., Nit-ac.*

left side, better lying on left side: *Sang.*

left side, worse lying on left side: *Eup-perf., Phos., Puls., Lach., Merc-s.* (breathing).

left side, worse lying on left side with respiration, but worse lying on right side with cough: *Merc-s.*

lying aggravates headaches, better sitting half propped: *Bell., Eup-perf., Gels.*

lying, better for lying on something hard, may lie on the floor: *Rhus-t.*

lying, lies with head back: *Ant-t.* (cough), *Bell.* (headache), *Hep-s.* (cough).

motion aggravates initially, continued motion relieves, over-exertion aggravates: *Rhus-t.*

motion aggravates vomiting: *Bry., Verat-a.*

motion aggravates (this may include talking, laughing, sneezing, eating): *Ant-t., Bell., Bry., Chel., Eup-perf.* (spine), *Gels., Nux-v.* (makes chillier).

motion aggravates, better for rest, worse for stooping and worse exertion: *Bry.*

motion makes him feel chillier: *Nux-v.*

motion, better gentle continuous motion, although generally worse for motion: *Gels.*

motion, better for motion, walking, stretching: *Pyrog.*

motion, better for moving gently around: *Gels., Puls.*

motion, paces up and down, goes from bed to bed, or total prostration: *Ars-a.*

motion, stitching pain independent of motion: *Kali-c.*

motionless: *Apis.*

painful side, better lying painful side, better pressure: *Bry.*

painful side, worse lying on painful side: *Phos.*

restlessness: *Acon., Apis, Ars-a., Bell., Mur-ac.* (at first), *Rhus-t.*

right side, worse lying on right side: *Crot-h., Kali-c., Merc-s.* (cough).

sits holding chest with cough: *Bry., Eup-perf., Nat-s.*

sits up to cough: *Ant-t., Ars-a.* (for breathing mainly), *Bry., Hep-s., Puls., Pyrog.*

sitting ameliorates pain: *Chel.*

sitting, better sitting half propped with headache particularly: *Bell., Gels., Eup-perf.*

sitting, cough better sitting up and generally worse for motion: *Ant-t.*

standing aggravates: *Sulph.*

stooping aggravates: *Bry.*

Prostration: *Apis* (stupor), *Ars-a., Ars-i., Bapt., Camph., Carb-ac., Gels., Mur-ac., Phos., Verat-a.*

Side: see also **Pneumonia**.
right, worse right side: *Apis, Bell., Chel., Crot-h., Merc-s., Sang.*
worse left side: *Lach., Rhus-t.*
worse left side, or worse left to right side: *Lach.*
Skin: see also **Face**.
bleeding through pores of skin, blood boils: *Crot-h.*
bluey, dusky red or purple discolouration: *Bapt., Lach.*
cellulitis, shingles, urticaria: *Rhus-t.*
cold and blue, bruised and marbled, with hot or cold perspiration: *Carb-v.*
cold, icy cold: *Camph., Carb-v., Verat-a.*
cracks corners mouth, eyes, anus: *Nit-ac.*
fever blisters and cold sores: *Rhus-t.*
dry: *Ars-a., Ars-i., Sulph.*
itching and dry, dry scalp and hair: *Ars-a.*
itching and redness anywhere: *Sulph.*
itching worse for warmth of bed: *Merc-s., Sulph.*
itching and burning: *Carb-ac.*
livid spots on body and limbs, burning heat, particularly on face, measles like eruption, urticaria, gangrenous sores, putrid ulcers: *Bapt.*
moist with easy sweating which does not relieve: *Merc-s.*
nettlerash: *Apis.*
puffy swellings œdema: *Apis.*
pustular eruptions: *Ant-t., Hep-s.*
pustular eruptions with cough: *Ant-t.*
pustular eruptions worse for touch: *Hep-s.*
red circumscribed blotches: *Sang., Sulph.*
sensitive to slightest touch and much worse for touch on right side of body: *Crot-h.*
sloughing of dead skin: *Crot-h.*
sore and red from acrid discharges: *Ars-a., Ars-i.*
wounds bleed a lot even if small, bleed easily: *Phos.*
Sleep:
better for a nap: *Nux-v., Phos.*
better for short naps, vivid dreams of fire and haemorrhage: *Phos.*
dreams of fire and blood: *Phos.*
dreams of great exertion: *Rhus-t.*
falls asleep while talking to you: *Bapt.*
fears going to sleep because of nightmares: *Bapt.*
jerks during: *Apis., Bell.*
jerks during, frightful visions on closing eyes: *Bell.*
waking around 3 am and cannot get back to sleep, better for a nap: *Nux-v.*
waking between 2 am and 4 am: *Kali-c.*

worse straight after sleep, worse on waking: *Apis., Lach.*
sleepiness and drowsiness with condition: *Ant-t., Apis.*
sleeplessness, with cold limbs: *Camph.*
sleepy, but cannot sleep: *Crot-h.*
sleepy, very sleepy: *Carb-ac.*

Stools:
black and involuntary: *Camph., Pyrog.*
black or brown, smelly: *Pyrog.*
black, dark, smelly, thin, bloody: *Bapt.*
black, thin, smelly, white, or like coffee grounds: *Crot-h.*
bloody: *Ant-t., Bapt., Crot-h., Ipec., Lach., Merc-s., Phos.*
bloody, white, weakness after: *Phos.*
changeable: *Puls.*
cream or green: *Gels.*
diarrhœa, autumn and hot weather, worse in: *Bapt.*
diarrhœa, drives out of bed in morning: *Sulph.*
diarrhœa, exhausting: *Phos.*
diarrhœa, from fright, nerves or bad news: *Gels.*
diarrhœa, from nervous anticipation: *Arg-n., Gels.*
diarrhœa, watery: *Ars-a., Ars-i.*
diarrhœa, with pneumonia: *Ant-t.*
frothy: *Ipec.*
green: *Acon., Ant-t., Crot-h., Gels., Merc-s.*
large, copious, much straining, violent: *Verat-a.*
large, dry hard: *Bry.*
pain, cutting and splinter pains after passing: *Nit-ac.*
pain, ineffectual and frequent urging: *Nux-v.*
pain, urging to pass stool with every pain: *Nux-v.*
painless, involuntary: *Pyrog.*
shreddy: *Carb-ac., Lach.*
smelly: *Bapt., Carb-ac., Crot-h., Lach., Merc-s., Pyrog.*
smelly, bloody, greenish, slimy, with straining: *Merc-s.*
smelly, brown or black: *Pyrog.*
smelly, thin, bloody, with straw-like shreds and particles: *Lach.*
smelly, thin, dark, bloody: *Bapt.*
watery diarrhœa: *Ars-a., Ars-i.*
white, cream: *Crot-h., Gels., Phos.*

Swallowing: see also **Throat.**
as if lump in throat: *Gels., Lach.*
as if lump in throat that cannot be swallowed: *Gels.*
can only swallow liquids, gags on food: *Bapt.*
cold things easier to swallow than hot: *Lach.*

difficult generally: *Carb-ac., Kali-c.*
difficult to swallow liquids: *Ant-t., Lach.*
difficult to swallow solids: *Crot-h., Rhus-t.*
empty swallowing worse, swallowing liquids difficult, easier swallowing food: *Lach.*

Sweats:
bloody and smelly, cold sweats: *Crot-h.*
easily: *Kali-c., Nit-ac.*
easily sweaty, chronically very sweaty: *Kali-c.*
easily, then catches cold from it: *Nit-ac.*
hot sweats although frozen: *Carb-v.*
on single parts, or one side only: *Sulph.*
profuse but it does not relieve: *Hep-s., Merc-s., Pyrog., Sulph.*
profuse night sweats: *Ars-i., Sulph.*
profuse, with all conditions: *Ant-t., Verat-a.*
profusely: *Ant-t., Ars-i., Kali-c., Merc-s., Verat-a.*
smelly: *Bapt., Crot-h., Merc-s., Nit-ac., Pyrog.*

Thirst and **Thirstlessness:** see **Digestion.**

Throat: see **Mouth**, see also **Swallowing.**
cold drinks ameliorate: *Apis., Lach.*
dry: *Bell., Bry.*
dry and hot with spasm in larynx, better for warm drinks, worse on right side, swollen shiny red tonsils: *Bell.*
dry constricted burning and stinging: *Acon.*
inflamed red, shiny, puffy, swelling like a bag of water: *Apis.*
inflamed, cold drink aggravates: *Bell., Hep-s.*
inflamed, cold drink ameliorates, but not thirsty: *Apis.*
inflamed, early stages: *Acon., Bell., Ferr-p.*
inflamed, red, shiny: *Acon., Apis., Bell., Ferr-p.*
left side worse, or left then right side, pain better for cold drinks, may be purple in colour: *Lach.*
liquids, can only swallow liquids, gags on food. Painless inflamed throat. Ulcers: *Bapt.*
lump, as if a lump in throat: *Gels., Lach.*
lump, as if a lump there which cannot be swallowed: *Gels.*
pain, burning from coughing: *Pyrog.*
pain, burning relieved by warm drinks: *Ars-a.*
pain, constricted: *Acon., Crot-h., Lach.*
pain, from throat to ear: *Gels., Hep-s., Merc-s., Nux-v.*
pain, rough and raw: *Merc-s., Rhus-t.*
pain, rough and tickling with stitches into ear: *Nux-v.*
pain, scratching like an apple core on throat: *Merc-s.*

pain, sharp, scratchy: *Hep-s., Merc-s., Nit-ac.*
pain, spasm: *Bell.*
pain, splinter-like: *Hep-s., Nit-ac.*
red, shiny puffy swelling like a bag of water: *Apis.*
swallowing difficult: *Ant-t., Crot-h., Kali-c., Lach.*

Time/Speed:

a cold travels fast from head to lungs, i.e. in a few hours or even minutes, but a fever comes on over a few days: *Bry.*
childhood and old age: *Ant-t.*
cough worse while eating and drinking: *Bry.*
early stages of fever or chill: *Acon., Bell., Camph., Ferr-p., Oscill.*
headaches start in morning and increase to noon then diminish: *Sang.*
later stages of a cold: *Hep-s.*
later stages of a cough: *Ant-t.*
older people often need this remedy more: *Ant-t., Carb-v., Verat-a.* (lungs).
periodicity: *Crot-h., Eup-perf., Sang.*
slow onset: *Bry.* (fever), *Gels., Puls.*
slow onset, but goes suddenly: *Puls.* (pains).
sudden onset: *Acon., Apis, Bapt.* (prostration), *Bell., Bry.* (cough), *Carb-ac.* (pains), *Ferr-p., Phos.* (prostration).
sudden onset, pains go suddenly too: *Bell., Carb-ac.*
worse 2 am, 3 am or 5 am: *Kali-c.*
worse 3 am or 3 pm: *Bell.*
worse 3 am: *Bell., Kali-c., Nux-v., Sang.*
worse early morning: *Hep-s., Nux-v.*
worse 4 am or 5 am: *Ant-t.* (cough), *Nat-s.*
worse 4 am to 6 am: *Ferr-p.*
worse 7 am to 9 am, or periodically such as every 3rd day or every 4th day: *Eup-perf.*
worse 9 am or 9 pm, in evening: *Acon.*
worse 11 am, an hour or so before lunch: *Sulph.*
worse 4 pm: *Apis.*
worse 4 pm for cough: *Ant-t.*
worse 4 pm in chill: *Puls.*
worse dusk: *Phos., Puls.*
worse evening: *Acon., Carb-v., Puls., Phos.*
worse midnight or noon: *Ars-a.*
worse night: *Acon., Merc-s., Sang.*
worse waking: *Apis, Bapt., Lach.*

Touch and Pressure:

aggravates: *Acon., Ant-t., Bapt., Bell., Hep-s., Lach., Merc-s., Mur-ac., Nux-v., Nit-ac., Sang.* (right side of body).

ameliorates: *Apis.* (head only), *Bry.* (but worse light touch), *Ipec., Phos., Pyrog., Puls., Rhus-t., Sang.* (bores head into pillow in headache).

better for massage: *Phos., Rhus-t.*

better lying on hard surface, e.g. floor, better for rubbing and massage: *Rhus-t.*

held, wants to be held as is shaking and trembling: *Gels.*

holds/supports chest with cough: *Eup-perf., Bry., Nat-s.*

touch aggravates, worse for light touch, better for pressure: *Bry.*

Tremors:

and weakness: *Ant-t.* (jaw), *Gels., Merc-s.*

Urine:

burning and smarting as it passes: *Apis.*

increases as headache gets better: *Gels.*

profuse: dark, and frequent: *Bell.*

scanty and high colour: *Apis.*

smelly, very smelly: *Bapt., Nit-ac., Pyrog.*

strong and smelly, feels cold as it passes: *Nit-ac.*

sugar in, blood in: *Phos.*

Voice: see **Cough/lungs**, hoarse.

Vomit and vomiting: see **Digestion.**

Weakness:

extreme prostration, collapse: *Ant-t., Apis, Ars-a., Bapt., Camph., Carb-v., Gels., Kali-c., Verat-a.*

Weather, Body Temperature, Reactions to:

air, cold air and draughts aggravate: *Hep-s., Rhus-t.*

air, damp air aggravates: *Carb-v., Ipec., Nat-s.*

air, damp air ameliorates: *Acon., Hep-s.*

air, desire for fresh air for lungs, ameliorates breathing: *Ars-a., Ars-i., Bapt., Carb-v., Ipec., Puls.*

air, desire for, even though very cold: *Carb-v.*

air, open air aggravates: *Hep-s., Nux-v.*

air, open air aggravates except for lungs: *Ars-a., Bapt.*

air, stomach and head better for cool open air, but cough worse dry air and also generally worse damp, wet and open air: *Crot-h.*

autumn and spring aggravate: *Ant-t., Bapt.*

chills in back and shivering: *Eup-perf., Gels.*

cold air aggravates: *Eup-perf., Hep-s., Merc-s., Nit-ac., Nux-v., Pyrog., Rhus-t., Verat-a.*

cold air aggravates and hot weather aggravates: *Nit-ac.*

cold ameliorates, worse heated: *Apis, Bry.*

cold and heat aggravate, sensitive to both: *Bapt., Merc-s.*
cold applications ameliorate: *Ferr-p.*
cold body but has hot head: *Gels.*
cold, blue with cold: *Carb-v.*
cold body, frozen, but head better for cold cool air: *Ars-a.*
cold, breath, tongue, limbs, all cold, whole body icy cold: *Camph.*
cold chills and creeping chilliness: *Merc-s.*
cold chills and/or heat run up and down back and shivering: *Gels.*
cold cool air relieves head and face symptoms but worsens cough: *Phos.*
cold dry windy weather aggravates: *Acon., Ars-i., Hep-s.*
cold, icy cold, worse anything cold, except cough which is better for cold: *Verat-v.*
cold, icy cold, but does not want covering up: *Camph., Carb-v.*
cold people: *Ars-a., Camph., Carb-v., Nat-s., Nux-v., Phos., Verat-a.*
cold to hot aggravates, hot to cold aggravates: *Phos.*
cold, uncovering aggravates: *Ars-a., Bell., Hep-s., Nux-v., Rhus-t.*
cold weather aggravates: *Eup-perf.* (extreme cold), *Kali-c., Merc-s., Pyrog.*
cold wet windy weather aggravates: *Bell., Rhus-t.*
cold when ill but usually warm person: *Puls.*
cold wind aggravates: *Acon., Ars-i., Bapt.*
cold worsens cough and sore throats, but relieves head and face symptoms: *Phos.*
cool air ameliorates: *Acon., Bry., Carb-v., Lach., Puls., Sang., Sulph.*
cool open air ameliorates stomach and head, but cough worse dry air although generally worse damp, wet and open air: *Crot-h.*
cough worse warm room but generally icy cold and better for warmth: *Verat-a.*
covering up aggravates: *Acon., Carb-v., Camph., Mur-ac.*
damp aggravates generally: *Crot-h., Ipec., Mur-ac., Nat-s., Pyrog.*
damp aggravates generally, also wet and open air, but cool open air ameliorates stomach and head, and cough worse dry air: *Crot-h.*
damp air ameliorates: *Acon., Hep-s.*
damp cold aggravates: *Ant-t., Mur-ac., Nat-s., Pyrog., Rhus-t.*
damp cold aggravates, spring and autumn aggravate, warmth and over heating aggravate: *Ant-t.*
damp heat, humid weather, mild winters aggravate, hot weather aggravates: *Gels.*
damp living conditions aggravate: *Ant-t., Nat-s.*
damp places aggravate, changes to wet weather aggravate: *Nat-s.*
draughts aggravate: *Bell., Kali-c., Rhus-t.*
dry air aggravates cough, although generally worse damp, wet and open air, stomach and head better for cool open air: *Crot-h.*
heat aggravates: *Gels., Nit-ac.*
heat and burning runs through remedy: *Acon.*
heat and warmth ameliorate burning pains: *Ars-a.*

heat, warmth, dry weather and winter weather aggravate: *Ipec.*
heated, getting over heated aggravates: *Ant-t., Bry., Merc-s., Puls.*
hot sun, exposure to, aggravates: *Acon., Bell., Gels., Verat-v.*
hot to cold aggravate, and cold to hot aggravates: *Phos.*
thunderstorms and lightning aggravate: *Phos., Rhus-t.* (mainly before storms).
uncovering ameliorates usually, although is cold, icy cold: *Camph., Carb-v.*
warm air aggravates, warm room aggravates: *Acon., Apis., Bry., Carbo-v., Ipec., Puls., Sulph., Verat-a.* (cough only).
warmth, heat and hot bath ameliorate: *Pyrog., Rhus-t.*
wet cold windy weather aggravates: *Bell., Rhus-t.*

Section Three

Homœopathic Materia Medica for Bird Flu

As mentioned previously, a homœopathic proving is a summary of all the symptoms produced when a remedy is tested on healthy people. The symptoms build up a picture of each remedy, and since *like is curing like* with homœopathic treatment, it follows that the remedy pictures are also descriptions of the symptoms each remedy can cure. A Materia Medica is a summary of these symptom pictures. This Materia Medica concentrates on the fever and chill, sweats, limb and back pains, digestive conditions, lung problems, throat and eye problems, and general weakness which are known to be important symptoms of flu generally, and Bird flu in particular. In a normal Materia Medica, covering **all** conditions and symptoms, the remedy pictures are **much** more extensive and detailed, but this is not required for the purposes of this book. [For instance there are many other remedies for earaches or severe throat conditions which often occur **without** flu or pneumonia-like symptoms. These can be found in *Homœopathy: the Modern Prescriber*, where they are described in more detail.] ***Remedies are only in this book if they are strongly part of a remedy picture relevant to flu, Bird flu or pneumonia.***

Using the Materia Medica

1. Causation does not refer to contact with the Bird flu virus, but to additional reasons why a particular person may be more susceptible to it at the time; obviously there has to have been contact with Bird flu.
2. *The symptoms written in italics in this Materia Medica are the most important ones and are the key features for each remedy picture. These are mainly the ones which are included in the Repertory.*

ACONITE

Main Indications *Acute sudden onset, inflammations, congestions, fevers, colds. Early stages of these particularly. Hot, burning, red and dry. Fright.*

Causation *Fright; exposure to cold, dry, windy weather or very hot dry weather.*

Mentals *Intense fear, restlessness and anxiety with all complaints, whether serious complaints or not;* frantic with fear and/or with the intensity of the pains. *May think they are going to die.* (See Ars-a.) *Can be delirious.*

Appearance/Head/Face/Eyes/Ears/Nose Appearance Usually *robust people when well.* *Head feels heavy, pulsating, hot and bursting, worse rising up.*

Eyes watering, eyelids swollen hard and red. Photophobia. *Contracted pupils.*

Face anxious and red which turns pale on rising up or on sitting up, and may alternate between being pale and red. (See Ferr-p.) One cheek may be hot and red and the other pale. Nose is dry and acutely sensitive to smell, pain at root of nose, *dry nose, or blocked up, or dry with slight watery discharge.* Nose may bleed.

Mouth/Throat *Throat dry, constricted, burning and stinging.* Tongue swollen tip which tingles, may have white coating.

Digestion/Appetite *Abdomen is worse for touch. Colic pain with restlessness. Stools green. Vomiting with fear, profuse sweat and increased urination.*

Appetite *Intense thirst* for cold drinks/water, but preferring bitter drinks such as beer. Worse for milk.

Cough/Lungs *Hoarse, croupy, dry cough, difficult breathing, short of breath, worse at night and after midnight, at 9 am or 9 pm. Croup with fever. Palpitations with anxiety, with pains in left shoulder. Pulse full hard tense and bounding.* Pneumonia, worse left lung and upper left lung. Expectoration may be bloody.

Extremities/Back *Numb and tingling, hot hands and cold feet.* Bright red hypothenar eminence (fleshy bit on inside of palm below little finger) on either hand. Pulse, either full and hard or hardly noticeable.

Fever/Chill *High fever with waves of coldness passing through them. In heat is better for uncovering. Restlessness. Dryness. Very thirsty through all stages of fever.* Hungry. When the fever breaks they are better for sweating. *Gastric fever.*

Pain Type Intense, *burning, dryness* running through this remedy picture; dry croupy cough, dry eyes, worse for cold, dry, windy weather, hot, dry inflammations. Numbness and tingling.

Touch/Pressure Worse touch and pressure.

Position/Motion *Very restless, tosses and turns.*

Light/Dark/Noise Eyes worse for light and *pupils contracted.* Generally worse for noise.

Weather/Body Temperature/Reactions Worse for warmth and heat *and better uncovering, better for open air and better keeping cool*; the acute illness is often *caused by exposure to cold, dry, windy weather.*

Time/Speed *Sudden onset always; the early stages of inflammations and acutes*; worse in the evening, *about 9 pm particularly,* and 9 am, and worse at night and after midnight.

Relationship to other remedies Compare Bapt. and Pyrog. in high fevers with sudden onset. Bell. and Ferr-p. for early stages. Puls. and Camph. better for uncovering. Gels., effects of shock, fright and bad news.

ANTIM. TART.

Main Indications Particularly indicated during *childhood and old age. May be very weak.* Collapse. *Great accumulation of mucus in the chest which is nearly impossible to expectorate. Cough with pustular eruptions. Drowsiness, sleepiness, weakness and sweats with all complaints.* Nausea is better for vomiting. *Pneumonia.*

Causation *Damp living conditions.* Effects of anger and vexation. Vaccination.

Mentals Irritable, easily annoyed or apathetic. Worse for touch but children may cling to those around them and want to be carried. Crying and whining. *Cough is worse if the person is angry.* Can be delirious.

Appearance/Head/Face/Eyes/Ears/Nose *Cold blue face covered with cold sweat, with incessant quivering of chin and lower jaw.* (Gels.) There may be a *blue/blackish/grey look around the mouth, lips, nostrils* and/or eyes. Flapping of nostrils. Ulcerated nostrils. Nosebleed and spongy bleeding gums.

Mouth/Throat *Tongue coated pasty thick white*, with red edges or streaks. Cannot really swallow liquids. Gums bleed.

Digestion/Appetite Usually *no thirst, or thirst for cold water little and often.* (Ars-a.) *Desires apples, fruits, acids. Nausea, retching and vomiting, nausea in waves.* Nausea may be better for vomiting. *Diarrhœa in pneumonia* and eruptive diseases. Stools may have mucus, be grass green, or bloody.

Cough/Lungs *Rattling of much mucus but with very little expectoration. Short of breath, coughing and gasping, feels as if suffocating. Chest is full of mucus but less and less is raised. Chest fills up with mucus threatening paralysis of lungs. Pneumonia. Lies with head back in lung disorders. Coughs when angry. Cough is worse at 4 am. Must sit up to cough.*

Extremities/Back *Violent pain in sacrolumbar area.* As if a heavy weight was hanging on the end of coccyx. Hands tremble.

Skin Pustular eruptions with cough.

Fever/Chill *Clammy with profuse sweat all over. Gastric fever, septic fever.*

Discharges *Clammy sweat, profuse.*

Touch/Pressure Worse touch.

Position/Motion *Cough is better sitting up.* Generally is worse for motion.

Weather/Body Temperature/Reactions Worse spring and autumn, *worse for damp*, worse for cold, *worse overheating and worse warmth, e.g. warm room and wraps.*

Time/Speed Usually required in later stages of a cough. Cough worse at 4 pm. Childhood and old age.

Sleep *Drowsiness and sleepiness with all complaints.*

Relationship to other remedies Nausea is as intense as with Ipec. but with Ant-t. it is less persistent and relieved by vomiting.

APIS

Main Indications *Puffy swellings, œdema or swelling like a bag of water.* This is not a main pneumonia remedy nor one for influenza particularly, but it can be indicated for septic fevers, if the remedy picture fits the symptoms, and for meningitis.

Causation *Meningitis, bites and stings, suppressed eruptions.*

Mentals *Extremely restless or slow and dull, or in a stupor. Prostration. Fussy and tidy, or clumsy and awkward. Worse if disturbed. Sudden sharp cries in delirium. Weeping, whining and jealous.*

Appearance/Head/Face/Eyes/Ears/Nose *Eyes Hot tears, swollen puffy eyelids, bloodshot and inflamed, sharp pains. Photophobia. Nose Red and swollen at tip. Headache Rolls the head from side to side with the pain, pressing into the pillow. Stabbing pains make them shriek.*

Mouth/Throat *Red shiny puffy throat better for cold drinks. Lips can be swollen.*

Digestion/Appetite *Usually thirstless. May want sour things or milk.*

Cough/Lungs *Dry cough, panting breathing, breathing difficult.*

Urine Scanty and high colour, *burning and smarting pains.*

Skin *Nettlerash, œdema, stinging. Puffy swellings.*

Fever/Chill *Burning during heat but chilly if moves. Chill in afternoon, about 4 pm, worse if moves and worse for heat. Septic fever.*

Pain Type *Burning, stinging and prickling.*

Side *Right.*

Touch/Pressure *Pressure and touch aggravate. Head can be better for pressure.*

Position/Motion *Either extremely restless or else motionless.*

Weather/Body Temperature/Reactions *Worse for heat and anything hot and better for cold cool things.*

Time/Speed *Sudden onset and worse after a sleep. Worse at 4 pm.*

Sleep *Sudden starting in sleep. Strong desire to sleep.* Worse after sleep.

Relationship to other remedies Incompatible: Rhus-t. It follows Bry. well.

ARGENT. NIT.

This remedy is not indicated for the wider picture of Bird flu but it is here because it is a *main conjunctivitis remedy* and may be indicated briefly during the course of the disease. However, you should always choose the remedy which fits the patient most **as a whole** as much as you can. Below is just a very brief description of the eye and throat symptoms.

Eye *Profuse, bland, thick, discharge from eye which may be cream, or green, or yellow. The whites of the eye are usually red or pink* and slightly swollen. These symptoms are very similar to the Pulsatilla conjunctivitis symptoms.

Throat *Splinter-like pains. Thick mucus.*

ARSENICUM ALBUM

Main Indications *Prostration and sinking of strength. Complete exhaustion. Suffering seems out of proportion to the actual symptoms. Vomiting and diarrhœa at the same time.*

Causation Eating watery fruit, drinking dirty water or eating dirty vegetables, particularly cold food and drink. Eating bad meat. Over-exertion and overheating. High altitudes, lack of oxygen.

Mentals *Extreme anxiety and restlessness. Fastidious*, critical and despair of recovery. *Fear of death.* (Acon.) Cannot stand any kind of disorder. *Very much worse alone. Can be delirious.*

Appearance/Head/Face/Eyes/Ears/Nose Face pale, yellow, sunken, shrivelled and old-looking, even if they are young. Look deathly pale. *Needle-like burning pains. Sit hugging the fire as very much worse for cold, but also will want the window open for fresh air. Sore, red skin from any discharges which are always acrid.* Itching scalp, *dry skin* and hair. Eyes *Severe photophobia, burning eyes with hot acrid tears.* Conjunctivitis, but discharge is acrid and thin. Nose thin watery excoriating discharge.

Mouth/Throat Burning pains which are better for warm drinks. Smelly breath, bleeding gums. Mouth ulcers.

Digestion/Appetite Burning *thirst but only takes sips at a time*; never drinks the whole mug in one go. Craves very cold water which may *vomit again immediately*; better for sips of warm water. Food poisoning usually from eating watery fruits, dirty water or vegetables and occasionally from eating bad meat. *Loathes, and has nausea at, the sight and smell of food. Burning pains anywhere including rectum.* Violent *cramping pains* in abdomen. *Diarrhœa watery, diarrhœa and vomiting at the same time, with either flu or food poisoning. Gastric fever.* Enlarged liver.

Cough/Lungs *Darting pain through upper third of right lung, burning or coldness in chest.* Gangrene of lungs. Yellow spots on chest. *Short of breath, must sit up, dry cough after drinking, expectoration frothy and scanty. All symptoms worse around, or soon after, midnight and midday.* Pneumonia.

Extremities/Back Restless and cold.

Skin *Dry. Sore, raw, red skin from acrid discharges.*

Fever/Chill *Septic fevers, coldness in spots, complete exhaustion, waves of icy coldness or intense burning heat, or externally cold and internally hot and burning. As if icy water or burning water running through veins. Gastric fever.*

Pain Type *Burning pains and cramping pains which are better for heat.*

Discharges *Any discharges are usually thin, acrid, excoriating and burning and will make the skin sore. Putrid and smelly discharges.*

Position/Motion *Extreme restlessness. Better moving and walking about. May even go from bed to bed, or pace up and down. There is also extreme prostration and exhaustion.*

Weather/Body Temperature/Reactions *Cold people, icy cold when ill, better* *wrapped up and close to the fire. However, they also crave fresh air, so despite being very chilly will insist on having the window wide open with the fire on. Burning pains are also better for heat and hot applications.*

Time/Speed *Worse soon after or around midnight and sometimes at midday as well.* There is very sudden sinking of strength and *prostration,* even from fairly trivial causes. Pulse faster in the morning.

Relationship to other remedies Complementary Carb-v., Phos.

ARSENICUM IODATUM

Main Indications *Corrosive, burning discharges. Prostration, pneumonia, pneumonia that fails to clear up.*

Appearance/Head/Face/Eyes/Ears/Nose *Burning acrid discharge from eyes, burning, acrid, excoriating discharge from nose, chronic nasal catarrh which burns.*

Digestion/Appetite *Chronic watery diarrhœa.*

Cough/Lungs *Pneumonia which does not clear up*, dry hacking cough, difficult expectoration, or yellowy green expectoration.

Skin Red and sore from the acrid discharge. *Scaly dry skin.*

Fever/Chill *Drenching night sweats.*

Pain Type *Burning from acrid discharge.*

Discharges *Discharges cause burning. Chronic acrid discharges cause burning of area they come from and over which they go. Profuse, thick, gluey, yellow, or thin discharges, but always acrid. Parts get red and sore. Drenching night sweats.*

Weather/Body Temperature/Reactions Better for open air, worse for dry foggy windy cold weather.

Relationship to other remedies Complementary to Phos.

BAPTISIA

Main Indications *Septic conditions of the blood, sick feeling all over, epidemic influenza. Prostration. Flu.*

Mentals *Thinks he is broken or double and tosses about the bed trying to get the pieces together. Cannot collect himself, confusion. Extremely restless.* Stupor, *falls asleep while speaking*, confused as if drunk. Wild wandering feeling in head. Delusion there is a smell of burnt feathers. Very drowsy. Fears going to sleep because of nightmares. *Can be delirious.*

Appearance/Head/Face/Eyes/Ears/Nose *Face dark red, bluey red, or dusky, besotted look. Cracked bleeding lips.* Eyes have *heavy eyelids*, bleary. Worse for light. *Head feels heavy and numb* and large.

Mouth/Throat *Mouth putrid, smelly breathe. Ulcerated. Can only swallow liquids. Tongue feels burned,* and swollen, speech difficult. Tongue coated yellowish white, then *dry parched brown at centre,* cracked and ulcerated.

Throat Can only swallow liquids, gags at food. Painlessness of inflamed throat. Painless ulcers in throat.

Digestion/Appetite *Sinking feeling in stomach, nausea.* *Abdomen* *Sensitive in lower right region of abdomen with rumbling.* *Rectum* *Smelly thin, dark, bloody stools.* Smelly diarrhœa, dysentery, worse autumn and worse hot weather. *Gastric fever.*

Cough/Lungs *Sense of suffocation.* Desire air, lungs feel tight, breathing difficult, want open air.

Urine *Very smelly.*

Extremities/Back *Heaviness and aching muscles, extreme muscular soreness, bed feels too hard.* (Lach. and Pyrog.)

Skin Livid spots on body and limbs, burning heat in skin, worse on face, measles like eruption or urticaria, foul sores, putrid ulcers.

Fever/Chill *High fever, sudden onset. Septic fevers. Gastric fever.*

Pain Type *Sick feeling all over, bed feels too hard. Painlessness of inflamed or ulcerated throat.*

Discharges *All very smelly; spit, urine, stools and sweat.*

Touch/Pressure *Worse for pressure. Worse lying on painful part.*

Position/Motion Worse walking.

Light/Dark/Noise Eyes worse for light.

Weather/Body Temperature/Reactions Worse for cold wind, autumn and hot weather. Desire air.

Time/Speed Worse on waking. *Rapid prostration.*

Sleep *Falls asleep while speaking.*

Relationship to other remedies Follows well after Ars-a.

BELLADONNA

Main Indications *Acute inflammation, congestions and fevers (particularly early stages). Heat, burning, swelling, bright redness, shiny, dryness. Glands swollen and red. Worse for touch. Worse right side. Fast onset.*

Causation *Exposure to cold, wet weather, getting hot and sweaty from exertion and then cooling down suddenly.* Exposure to very hot sun; having hair washed/cut.

Mentals *Angry and irritable*, grumpy and difficult. They are *restless and hypersensitive to everything, such as noise, light, touch etc.* If the temperature goes really high there can be *delirium with a great deal of restlessness, fury and rages; they see monsters, and can be violent then, with shrieking and biting.*

Appearance/Head/Face/Eyes/Ears/Nose Head has *throbbing hammering headache, better lying slightly propped* or bending head back, *worse light, noise, jar, at 3 am and 3 pm. Shiny, bright red, hot and dry inflammations and swellings.* Face *may be fiery red in fever.* Nose bleeds with red face. Eyes may be red, *pupils are dilated and their eyes are worse for light.* Ears may be inflamed and painful.

Mouth/Throat *Strawberry-like tongue. Grinding teeth.* *Throat* *dry and hot, spasm in larynx. Throat pain better for warm drinks, often worse on right side. Red shiny throat, swollen tonsils worse on right. Hoarse voice.* Chewing motion.

Digestion/Appetite *Very thirsty, particularly for lemonade or cold water, although throat pain is usually better for warm drinks. Gastric fever.*

Cough/Lungs *Dry tickling cough worse in the night. Moaning at every breath, high piping voice, larynx very painful.*

Urine *Profuse, dark, frequent and turbid, and may be bloody.*

Extremities/Back *Cold limbs,* joints swollen and shining with red streaks radiating. They have cold extremities, weak and tottering gait, jerks and spasms in the limbs with a heavy paralytic feeling. The back can feel broken, with stiffness of the neck and back.

Fever/Chill *Usually has a very high temperature with hot head and cold limbs. May feel very chilly despite high fever, and need to be covered up. Burning pungent, steaming heat. May have no thirst during fever. Spasms in throat. Very thirsty, particularly for lemonade or cold water. Face is fiery red in fever. Gastric fever.*

Pain Type *Throbbing, pulsating, sharp, cutting, shooting, spasmodic or cramping. Acuteness of all senses to noise, light etc., all of which aggravate the patient.*

Side *Worse on right side.*

Touch/Pressure *Worse for slightest touch and worse for pressure.*

Position/Motion *Prefer to be lying half propped against the pillows* or bending head backwards particularly if they have a headache. Worse for motion, worse for jarring, worse hanging down the affected part. Very restless.

Light/Dark/Noise *Worse for noise and light.*

Weather/Body Temperature/Reactions Worse for cold, *can feel freezing inside even if their temperature is high, worse uncovering, worse for draughts*, better in warm room, better for closed windows. *Onset from exposure to cold, wet windy weather as well as from hot sun.* Patient is burning hot. Skin is red and dry but is probably damp and sweaty under the hair, under the clothes or bedclothes.

Time/Speed *Worse 3 am or 3 pm or starts round these times. Sudden onset.* Pains may come and go suddenly. Early stages of inflammations.

Sleep *Jerks during sleep. Sees frightful visions on closing eyes. Grinding teeth.*

BRYONIA

Main Indications *Worse for motion. Painful dry cough, worse for motion. Headache and pains better for pressure, worse for motion. Thirst for cold drinks. Dryness throughout remedy. Flu. Pneumonia.* Used to living well and usually is healthy and strong.

Causation Anger, fright, chagrin. Drinking very cold drinks in hot weather. Suppressed eruptions and discharges.

Mentals Wants to go home even though is at home. *Very irritable.* Anxiety about business. *Can be delirious.*

Appearance/Head/Face/Eyes/Ears/Nose Head pains worse for *motion, bursting and splitting. Must lie down with headache which is better for pressure.* Pain to left eye area, then back of head and then whole body. Face may be dark red. Nose bleeding (may be from suppression of menstruation). Chewing motion of jaws like Bell. but Bell. does not have very dry lips etc. Vertigo, faint and dizzy *worse for motion.*

Mouth/Throat *Mouth dry and parched, cracked lips, dry tongue and throat and extreme thirst, bitter taste.*

Digestion/Appetite *Thirst for large quantities of water, which ameliorates them. Bitter taste. Large, dry, hard stools. Nausea and faint when rising up, or on motion. Stomach, worse for touch, but better for hard pressure, as if a stone in stomach after food. Gastric fever.*

Cough/Lungs *Sharp, stitching pains. Very dry hard hacking painful cough, with extreme thirst; must sit up to cough although worse for motion; holds chest when coughing, worse eating or drinking, worse in warm room and worse for taking a deep breath.* Rusty expectoration, blood streaked and tough. *Pulse full and quick.* Pneumonia. Right lung worse. Cough may cause headache.

Extremities/Back *Joints red, swollen and hot. Stitching and tearing pain anywhere, worse for motion.*

Fever/Chill Chill with external coldness, stitching pains and dry cough. Hot head and red face. Dry burning heat in fever, easy profuse sweat when fever breaks. *Gastric fever. Septic fever.*

Pain Type *Stitching, tearing, like a knife, bursting (particularly headache).*

Discharges *Dryness throughout remedy.*

Touch/Pressure *Better for pressure, worse for light touch, better for lying painful side.*

Position/Motion *Worse for motion, better for rest, worse for stooping, worse for exertion. Sits up to cough.*

Weather/Body Temperature/Reactions Cold with hot head and red face, *better for cool air, cold things, worse becoming hot.*

Time/Speed *A head cold travels fast down to lungs, i.e. in a few hours, but fever generally comes on over a few days.*

CAMPHORA

Main Indications *Collapse. Icy cold but does not want to be covered. First stage of colds and flu. Desires cold things,* cold drinks and snacks.

Causation Shock, injury, operations, sunstroke. Vexation.

Mentals Wants company, wants care and attention during hot stage of fever. Anxious. *Can be delirious.*

Appearance/Head/Face/Eyes/Ears/Nose *Anxious look, bluish colour. Headache with flu, catarrh and sneezing, with occipital (back of head) throbbing pain, synchronous with pulse. Fleeting stitches in temples and eye orbits. Nose is cold and pinched looking and may have a persistent nosebleed.*

Mouth/Throat *Tongue cold. Breath is cold.*

Digestion/Appetite *Desires cold* drinks and snacks. Stools black and involuntary.

Cough/Lungs *Breath is very cold, and lungs feel cold.*

Urine Can only pass drops because of spasms and contractions at neck of bladder. Straining.

Extremities/Back *Extreme coldness. Insomnia with cold limbs.*

Fever/Chill *Icy coldness of whole body, shaking with cold but only wants to be covered during the hot stage.*

Pain Type *Bad cramps.*

Weather/Body Temperature/Reactions *Icy cold but does not want to be covered except during hot stage. Whole body is cold. Tongue is cold.*

Time/Speed *First stages of cold and flu.*

Sleep *Insomnia with cold limbs.*

Relationship to other remedies This remedy is strongly antidotal to other remedies and should not be kept close by other homœopathic remedies, so remember to keep it separately.

CARBOLIC ACID

Main Indications *Marked prostration, destructive septic conditions, foul discharges. Very sensitive to smell.* This is not a major remedy for pneumonia but it could be useful in some septic conditions (e.g. if organs are breaking down).

Causation *Allergic reactions* (bees, see Apis).

Mentals *Prostration*. Can be delirious.

Appearance/Head/Face/Eyes/Ears/Nose *Nose very sensitive to smells. Face pale around nose and mouth.*

Mouth/Throat *Very smelly breath. Can barely swallow.*

Digestion/Appetite Burping, nausea, vomiting and wind. *Burning from mouth to stomach. Can hardly swallow; regurgitation. Desire for stimulants. Shreddy stools, smelly stools.*

Skin *Burning and itching.*

Pain Type *Painlessness or burning sensations. Pains may come and go suddenly.*

Discharges *Very smelly and burning.*

Sleep *Very sleepy.*

Relationship to other remedies Follows Verat-a. well.

CARBO VEG.

Main Indications Often indicated for fat and old people. Lazy. *Affects veins and circulation. Icy cold, body goes blue. Desires fresh air, fanning, and windows to be open. Weakness with craving for cool air. Effects of a previous illness. Almost lifeless, weak and exhausted. Septic conditions, blueness and decomposition. Collapsed. Haemorrhages, dark blood oozing persistently for hours or days* (e.g. after shock of surgery).

Causation *Loss of fluids and/or a previous illness from which they have not fully recovered. Usually high living, rich food etc., and wine. Bad meat. Fatty food. Typhoid fever, yellow fever, cholera, malaria, and quinine abuse.*

Mentals Sluggish, slow, indifference, unhappy, lazy, easily frightened and startled. Can be delirious.

Appearance/Head/Face/Eyes/Ears/Nose *Head sore and hair falls out easily. Face has pinched blue look,* pimples, mottled cheeks and red nose, lips brown or black and cracked. *Nose bleeding daily with pale face. Body blue and icy cold. Blueness and decomposition.*

Mouth/Throat *Breath is cold and smelly.* Gums bleed.

Digestion/Appetite *Very windy and worse for rich food and wine. Distended abdomen, flatulent colic, averse to fat. Digestion slow, food putrefies, even worse after simplest food; burping, fullness and sleepiness.* Contractions in abdomen which is distended and pain extends to chest. Acrid corrosive moisture from rectum. Blue piles. *Gastric fever.*

Cough/Lungs *Must be fanned to get enough fresh air, cough with burning in chest,* spasmodic cough, asthma in elderly with blue skin, *much rattling mucus in chest,* expectoration with retching. Pneumonia. Thick, sticky, yellow, profuse expectoration. Some long coughing attacks. Contractions in abdomen which is distended and pain extends to chest. Hoarseness worse in the evenings.

Extremities/Back *Cold from knees downwards particularly.* Limbs go to sleep easily.

Skin Varicose ulcers. *Skin cold, blue, bruised and marbled, but has hot perspiration in septic conditions.*

Fever/Chill *Alternating chill and heat, icy coldness with burning in various parts too. Hot or cold perspiration. Pneumonia. Gastric fever. Septic fever.*

Pain Type Cold but with burning in chest. Distended abdomen.

Discharges *Odour fetid, skin cold and blue with a bruised, marbled appearance but can have hot perspiration with septic fever. Hot or cold perspiration. Haemorrhages dark blood, oozing.* Acrid discharges from rectum.

Weather/Body Temperature/Reactions *Desires fresh cold air, wants windows open, worse for warmth.* Worse damp. *Icy cold body, goes blue.*

Time/Speed Worse in evening and damp air. *Lack of reaction.* Older people.

CHELIDONIUM

Main Indications *Liver, pain inner angle right shoulder blade, yellow, jaundice, right sided.*

Mentals *Can be delirious.*

Appearance/Head/Face/Eyes/Ears/Nose *Yellow. Jaundice. Drowsy.*

Mouth/Throat Smelly breath.

Digestion/Appetite *Pain lower inner angle of right shoulder blade. Associated with liver problems. Jaundiced. Bilious. Wants only warm food and drink. Gastric fever.*

Cough/Lungs Cough loose and rattling but expectoration very difficult (Ant-t., Ipec.). *Deep pain in whole of right chest.* Pneumonia with digestive problems. Right upper lung worse.

Extremities/Back *Pain lower inner angle of right shoulder blade.* One foot cold the other hot.

Fever/Chill Fever and pneumonia. Gastric fever.

Pain Type *Shoots through stabbing like a knife, worse for motion.*

Side *Right side.*

Position/Motion *Worse for motion. Sits up with the pain, despite being worse for motion.*

Relationship to other remedies Complementary to Bry., Ars-a., Ipec., and Sulph.

CROTALUS HORRIDUS

Main Indications *Sloughing of skin. Septic conditions. Haemorrhages from every part of the body. (Yellow fever, cholera, plagues generally.) Low septic conditions. More right-sided. Liver affections, jaundice* (Lach. has septic conditions and fever but is left-sided).

Causation Fright, sun, lightning, alcohol, foul water, insect stings, sewage, vaccinations.

Mentals Easily tearful, agony and despair, confusion, perception clouded and memory impaired. *Can be delirious.*

Appearance/Head/Face/Eyes/Ears/Nose *Eyes and behind eyes have neuralgic pains, helps absorption of eye haemorrhages, eyes worse for light, particularly artificial light. Nose bleeding black blood and/or stringy blood.* Tip of nose blue and/or red. *Blood oozes from any orifice.*

Throat/Mouth Smelly breath, increased saliva (Merc-s.) and bloody saliva. Constricted stiff tongue and throat which impedes speech, tongue protrudes to the right, tongue small but feels swollen. Cannot swallow solids.

Digestion/Appetite *Liver pain, jaundice and haemorrhage.* Stitches, aching and coldness. Stomach worse for pressure of clothing (Lach.), vomiting of bile, food and/or blood, vomits if lies on right side, black or coffee ground type vomit. Very thirsty. *Bleeding from anus. Stools black, thin, smelly, like coffee grounds,* dark green or white.

Cough/Lungs Dry cough. Bloody sputum. Worse dry air.

Skin *Bleeding. Bloody sweat. Skin is sensitive particularly on right side of body. Worse for slightest touch to right side of body. Swelling of affected part. Blood boils.* Sloughing of skin.

Fever/Chill Bloody sweat, cold sweat. *Septic fever.*

Discharges *Bloody, coffee grounds, black, green, smelly. Blood oozes from any orifice.*

Side *Right-sided, worse lying on right side.*

Touch/Pressure *Right side of body very sensitive to touch.*
Position/Motion *Worse lying on right side.*
Weather/Body Temperature/Reactions Cough worse for dry air, although generally is worse for damp wet and open air; but stomach and head better for open air.
Time/Speed Periodicity.
Sleep Sleepy but cannot sleep.

EUP. PERF.
Main Indications *Backache, limb muscles ache, bones ache in particular, and are sore and feel broken.* Sore skin as well as bones and muscles, shivering and chills. Desires cold water but may vomit food, drink and bile. Headache with nausea, sore chest with cough.
Causation Being in extreme cold.
Appearance/Head/Face/Eyes/Ears/Nose Eyes *Eyeballs sore, extreme aching eyes.* (Gels.) Head *Pain at back of head, worse after lying down with sense of a weight in that area. Bilious sick headaches. Headache with nausea. Headache coming on during the chill, but worse during the sweat of the fever.*
Digestion/Appetite *Hiccough. Nausea worse for smell or sight of food. Thirst for cold water followed by shuddering and vomiting of bile, food and drink. Bilious sick headaches.* Gastric fever.
Cough/Lungs *Cough with soreness in chest,* must support chest with cough, *chronic loose cough worse at night. Hoarseness. Cannot lie on left side, difficult breathing with sweat.* Sore chest with cough.
Extremities/Back *Aching and soreness in limbs and back as if bones broken. Cannot move as it worsens the pain.* (Bry., opposite to Pyrog.) *Thirst, and soreness and aching of bones, precede the chill. Aching in arms and wrists, limbs and back.*
Fever/Chill *Chills in back and shivering. Worse for cold air. The chill is preceded by thirst and also soreness and pain in bones. Chill worse between 7 am and 9 am, and/or every third or fourth day.* Gastric fever.
Pain Type *Soreness internally, particularly of eyes and bones. Aching in bones, sore flesh and tearing muscles.*
Side Worse lying left side (lungs).
Position/Motion Better on hands and knees, better lying on face. *Cannot lie on left side. Cannot move as it worsens the pain.* Holds chest with cough.
Weather/Body Temperature/Reactions *Worse for cold air.*
Time/Speed *Worse 7-9 am, every 3rd or 4th day.*
Relationship to other remedies Bry., Chel.

FERRUM PHOS.
Main Indications *First stage of any inflammatory conditions. Catches cold easily. Anaemia.*

Causation Bad effects of checked sweat, mechanical injuries.

Mentals Not the restlessness of Acon., or Bell., nor the lethargy or weakness of Gels. *but is between the two extremes.*

Appearance/Head/Face/Eyes/Ears/Nose *Nosebleeds. Bloodshot eyes. Alternates between being flushed and pale.* Headaches relieved by cold flannel. *First stage of ear inflammation.*

Mouth/Throat Tonsils red and swollen, first stage of inflammation, laryngitis.

Digestion/Appetite *Vomits undigested food. Sour burping. Very thirsty.* (Phos.)

Cough/Lungs *Coughs up pure clear blood. Pneumonia. Dry cough.*

Fever/Chill *Early stages of fever, pneumonia. Not many indications.* Not as energetically sick as Bell., or Acon., nor as lethargic as Gels.

Discharges Bloody.

Weather/Body Temperature/Reactions *Better for cold applications.*

Time/Speed *Early stages of fevers, early stage of local inflammations.* Worse 4-6 am.

Relationship to other remedies Early stage of fevers and inflammations like Bell., Acon. and Camph.

GELSEMIUM

Main Indications *Aching, weakness and tremors particularly in muscles, limbs and back. Heaviness, drowsiness, lack of muscular co-ordination, even paralysis. Fevers accompanied by these symptoms. Drowsy, apathetic, dizzy and trembling. Heavy eyelids with bruising headache from the neck to head and forehead. Chill and heat. No thirst. Paralysis of various kinds. Never been well since flu. Chill up and down back.*

Causation *Hot climates, heat of sun, summer. Damp, hot, humid weather. Temporary anticipatory fears. Mild winters. Bad news. Fear of disease.*

Mentals Nervousness, temporary *anticipatory fears, e.g. of the disease, or else sinks into apathy. Shaking, trembling with fear.* Better alone, does not want anyone near them even if they are silent. Apathetic. Dazed. Dread of falling. *Can be delirious.*

Appearance/Head/Face/Eyes/Ears/Nose *Head pain bursting extends from neck over head to eyes and forehead; as head pain improves, urination increases. Pain in temple extending to ear. Band pain round head, or in occiput, (back of head). Headache better sitting propped up. Face hot flushed heavy stupefied look. Eyes ache. Droopy eyelids. Dizzy and blurred vision. Twitching of eye muscles. Shaking, trembling.* Hands tremble. Vertigo, dizzy *and blurred vision.*

Mouth/Throat *As if a lump in throat which cannot be swallowed, pain from throat to ear.* (Hep-s. and Merc-s.) Spasm in larynx. Dry mouth.

Digestion/Appetite May become thirsty during sweat only. Dry mouth and lips, but *no thirst. No thirst even during heat of fever. Diarrhœa from fright, bad news, or anticipation. Stools cream coloured or green. Gastric fever.*

Cough/Lungs Crowing inspiration, dry cough with sore chest, slow breathing, lung spasms. Heart Weak, slow pulse of old age. *Feels must keep moving or heart's action would cease.*

Extremities/Back *Chills and heat chase each other up and down back. Weak and trembling limbs. Muscular soreness and prostration in fever.*

Fever/Chill *Chills and heat chase each other up and down back. Wants to be held as is shaking so much. No thirst even during heat of fever.* May become thirsty during sweat. *Muscular soreness and prostration in fever.* Gastric fever.

Pain Type Aching, *heaviness*, soreness.

Discharges *Better for profuse urination, particularly the headache.* Generally better for sweating.

Position/Motion Worse for motion generally because of the extreme weakness. Worse for downward motion. Better continuous gentle motion. *Better sitting propped up particularly when they have a headache.*

Weather/Body Temperature/Reactions Generally worse for heat. *Worse in humid, damp, hot weather and mild winters.* Hot head with cold body. *Shivers of cold run up and down spine*, despite being hot and sweaty.

Time/Speed Slowish onset.

HEPAR SULPH.

Main Indications *Catarrhal, pus, touchy, splinter-like pains. Smelly.*

Causation *Cold dry wind.*

Mentals *Irritable and touchy in the extreme.* Can be delirious.

Appearance/Head/Face/Eyes/Ears/Nose Ears Pains are *sharp and scratchy* and may go from throat to ear; the ear may have a thick smelly, often yellow, discharge. Nose bleeds. Conjunctivitis, profuse purulent discharge, worse for touch and sensitive to air.

Mouth/Throat *Splinter-like pains* that are worse on swallowing; may feel like a crumb in the throat. Pains are *sharp and scratchy and may go from throat to ear. Pains are aggravated by touch and the patient prefers warm drinks to cold. Voice may be hoarse or lost with the throat symptoms.* Gums bleed.

Cough/Lungs *Cough at slightest uncovering or from cold air or cold food. Better in damp weather. Dry cough or more often loose and rattling;* has to sit up and may bend head back. Pneumonia.

Skin *Eruptions very sensitive to touch, suppurations and ulcers.*

Fever/Chill *Chilly from slightest draught.*

Pain Type *Splinter-like, sharp, darting, scratchy.*

Discharges *Thick and smelly. Sour smell. Profuse sweat; no relief from sweat.*

Touch/Pressure *Worse for touch, even very slight touch.*

Weather/Body Temperature/Reactions *Worse for cold and better for warmth. Worse from slightest draught or uncovering. Worse in dry weather, better for damp.*

Time/Speed *Worse in the early hours of the morning, later stages in colds.*

Relationship to other remedies Follows Acon. and Bell. well. Similarities with and compatible: Lach., Merc-s., and Nit-ac.

IPECAC.

Main Indications *Persistent nausea and vomiting which does not relieve. Continuous nausea. Bright red profuse haemorrhages, gushing. Clean or cleanish tongue, despite the vomiting and digestive problems.*

Causation Probably have a history of nosebleeds and of bleeding easily. May have a history of morphine or heroin addiction. Rich food. Quinine. From suppressed eruptions.

Mentals *Vexation, reserved displeasure.* Children yell, cry and are impossible to please. *Can be delirious.*

Appearance/Head/Face/Eyes/Ears/Nose Migraines with nausea and vomiting. Eyes inflamed red with conjunctivitis. Gushing tears with nausea. *Bleeds from mouth and nose (particularly aggravated by cough). Pale blue/grey round eyes and lips.* Small blister like eruptions on lips.

Mouth/Throat *Tongue clean despite digestive symptoms.* Hoarse voice.

Digestion/Appetite *Nausea no better for vomiting. Constant nausea. Pain round navel. Frothy bloody stools. Gastric fever. Thirstlessness.*

Cough/Lungs *Constriction in chest. Incessant and violent cough. Loose course rattle in chest without expectoration.* (Ant-t.) *Pneumonia. Bleeding from lungs.*

Fever/Chill Chill alternating with heat. Heat without thirst. Catarrhal and gastric fevers. Hands and feet drip cold sweat. *Chill is worse for warm room. Better for rest, better for cold drinks. Gastric fever.*

Pain Type *Pain round navel.*

Discharges *Bloody, bright red, gushing. Frothy stools.*

Touch/Pressure *Better for pressure.*

Weather/Body Temperature/Reactions Better for air, worse in winter, worse for dry weather, *worse for warmth*, worse for damp.

KALI CARB.

Main Indications *Sweats profusely, backache and weakness.*

Causation Bad effects of suppressions, suppressed eruptions in childhood diseases, pneumonia, colds, overstrain.

Mentals *Full of fears and over-active imagination, fear of ghosts etc. Hypersensitive to pain.* Can be delirious.

Appearance/Head/Face/Eyes/Ears/Nose *Nose stuffs up in warm room. Ulcerated nostrils.* Bloody nasal discharge.

Mouth/Throat *Swallowing difficult.*

Digestion/Appetite *Stomach as if full of water, sour belching, nausea.*

Cough/Lungs *Stabbing pains independently from respiration. Affects lower right side of chest particularly.* Cannot lie on right side (Bry. lies on affected side as is better for hard pressure). *Mucus rattling in chest with cough but difficult expectoration.* (Ant-t., Ipec.) *Chest is very sensitive. Pneumonia.*

Extremities/Back *Weak muscles of back and of limbs. Lower back very weak. Soles very sensitive.*

Fever/Chill *Pneumonia.* Internal burning in fever, or chilly but may have hot hands. Sweats on the least exertion. Sweats on parts that hurt.

Pain Type *Stabbing and stitching* (Bry.) *but these pains are also independent of respiration* (Bry. stitching pains are only with movement as Bry. is worse for movement). *Hypersensitive to pain.*

Discharges Sweats on least exertion and/or painful parts. *Profuse sweats.*

Side Worse on right side.

Position/Movement Worse lying on right side.

Weather/Body Temperature/Reactions *Worse in cold weather and worse draughts.* In fever has internal burning. Can be chilly but may have hot hands.

Time/Speed *Worse at 2 am, 3 am, or 5 am.*

Sleep *Waking between 2 am and 4 am.*

Relationship to other remedies Complementary to Carbo-v., and Nux-v.

LACHESIS

Main Indications *(1) Cannot stand wearing anything tight anywhere, worse for touch. Sensation of constriction (round neck and waist particularly). (2) Worse on left side or symptoms go from left to right side. (3) Worse after sleep. Symptoms wake him up. (4) Better for all discharges, worse for stopped discharge. (5) Bluish red or purple discolourations. Malignant and septic states. Flushes of heat. Sensation of lump in throat. Haemorrhages.*

Causation *Suppressed discharges anywhere. Jealousy, alcohol.*

Mentals *Delirium with trembling and confusion. Extreme loquacity, jealous and suspicious. Fears going to sleep because will be worse when wakes.*

Appearance/Head/Face/Eyes/Ears/Nose *Face swollen mottled and puffed purple blue. Pressure or burning on top of head. Nosebleeds on blowing nose.*

Mouth/Throat *Mouth ulcers and denuded spots, bluish purplish gums and easily bleeding. Bad smell. Left sided throat. Better for cold drinks.* Toothache extends to ears. *As if there is a lump in throat. Sensation of constriction of throat, worse for empty swallowing and worse for swallowing liquids.* As if a plug moves up and down throat with cough. *Sensation of suffocation and strangulation.*

Digestion/Appetite *Worse for anything tight round waist. Very smelly stool. Thin bloody stools, with shreds and particles like straw.* Stomach pain better for eating.

Cough/Lungs *Breathing difficult if has anything tight round throat, needs to take a deep breath, breathing almost stops on falling asleep.* As if a plug moves up and down throat with cough. *Sensation of suffocation and strangulation; worse covering mouth or nose. Oppression of chest.* Worse lying on left side. *Expectoration can be bloody. Septic lungs. Worse left lung.*

Fever/Chill *Heat on top of head in waves/flushes. Septic fevers. Pneumonia.*
Pain Type *Constriction. Pressing pain.*
Discharges *Septic and bleeds. Haemorrhages are thin and contain particles like straw.*
Side *Worse on left side, or symptoms go from left to right side.*
Touch/Pressure *Worse for anything tight anywhere.*
Position/Motion Worse lying on left side.
Weather/Body Temperature/Reactions *Better for cold air, better for open air, worse for hot drinks.*
Time/Speed *Worse for or after sleep.*

MERC. SOL. OR MERC. VIV.
Main Indications *Sensitive to both heat and cold. Tremors. Smelly discharges. Indecision.*
Mentals Constantly changing mind. *Indecision. Poor self confidence. Can be delirious.*
Appearance/Head/Face/Eyes/Ears/Nose *Face appears earthy or pale. Ears have thick yellow smelly discharge, and ear pains are worse for warmth of bed. Eyes have burning acrid discharge. Conjunctivitis with redness soreness of eyes. Pain in bones round the eye as well as in the eye in colds. Head pain as if bandaged, tension on scalp. Nose has rawness inside nostrils, ulcerated with swelling and decay of nasal bones; green smelly ulceration. Nosebleed with cough.*
Mouth/Throat *Tongue indented by teeth, furrowed lengthwise, yellow flabby with teeth indentations, sweet or metallic taste, very smelly breath. Spongy bleeding gums. Pain like an apple core scratching the throat. Smarting, raw or sore pain. Mouth has increased saliva, may dribble. Smelly breath. Thirsty despite profuse saliva. Ulcers. Pain from throat to ear.*
Digestion/Appetite *Desires cold drinks and beer, continuous hunger. Diarrhœa, bloody, greenish, slimy and smelly; straining. Gastric fever.*
Cough/Lungs Pain below right breast particularly through to back, worse for sneezing or coughing. *Smelly breathe always.* Cough in double bouts, dry at night, yellow green sputum by day, shortness of breath worse going upstairs or walking fast, breathing difficult worse for lying on left side but cough worse for lying on right side. Nosebleed particularly from violence of cough. Jaundice in pneumonia. Right lung worse.
Extremities/Back *Trembling limbs and hands. Tremors.*
Skin *Constantly moist, easy sweat but no better for it. Itching worse for warmth of bed.*
Fever/Chill *Sweats profusely but without relief. Creeping coldness. Worse when heated. Gastric fever. Septic fever.*
Pain Type *Burning and raw from acrid discharges.*
Discharges *Always very smelly, easy and profuse sweating but feels no better for it.*

Acrid and burning discharges; usually thick, smelly, yellow or green.

Side Cough worse lying on right side but breathing difficult lying on left side. *Can be more right sided.*

Touch/Pressure *Touch and pressure aggravate.*

Position/Motion Worse lying right side; cough worse lying right side, respiration difficult lying on left side.

Weather/Body Temperature/Reactions *Sensitive to heat and cold. Worse when heated. Creeping chilliness.*

Time/Speed *Worse in night.*

Relationship to other remedies Similar to Bell. and Hep-s. (particularly in throat sticking pain); like Puls., but with Puls. the nasal discharge is bland; like Nux-v. in coryza and sore throat, but Nux-v has a scraped feeling and Merc-s. is smarting, raw and sore. With stool/diarrhœa Nux-v. straining ceases after stool, but with Merc-s. there is a never get done feeling; Acon. has dysentery during hot days and cold nights. Ars-a. is better for heat of bed, worse for rest, but Merc-s. is worse for heat of bed and better for rest. Merc-s. has right or left sided shooting pains in different directions, in lungs; Chel. and Kali-c. affect lower lobe of right lung with stitches through to back.

MURIATIC ACID

Main Indications This is indicated for *septic fevers and prostration* more than flu and particularly if the digestive system is affected.

Mentals *Restlessness from pains and soreness. Moans or is silent.* Can be delirious.

Appearance/Head/Face/Eyes/Ears/Nose Face dark or glowing red. *Nosebleeds. Sneezing.* Rough lips, *cracked and scabby.*

Mouth/Throat Swollen and bleeding gums. Foul breath. *Sordes (brown crusty accumulations) on teeth and lips. Ulcerations of mouth. Dryness of mouth and throat.*

Digestion/Appetite Fullness and distension. Involuntary stools, not very painful. *Ulcerations.* Gastric fever.

Extremities/Back *Muscles exhausted.*

Urine Has to wait a long time for urine to pass. Passes stool at same time.

Skin Ulcerations.

Fever/Chill *Septic fevers, burning heat better for uncovering,* but limbs may be cold. Gastric fever.

Pain Type *Soreness causing restlessness but then leads to prostration. Burning pains.*

Discharges Haemorrhages.

Side *Vertigo worse lying on left side. Cannot lie on left side.*

Position/Motion *Restlessness at first but very exhausted so finds it difficult to move.*

Touch/Pressure Touch aggravates.

Weather/Body Temperature/Reactions Wet weather aggravates. Cold drinks or cold applications aggravate. Better uncovering.

Relationship to other remedies Compare Bapt. and Bry.

NATRUM SULPH.

Main Indications *Copious thick mucus. Wet, damp weather aggravates.*

Causation *Wet, damp weather. Head injuries.*

Mentals Sad and low, worse for listening to music.

Appearance/Head/Face/Eyes/Ears/Nose *Thick yellow nasal discharge with salty mucus. Nosebleeds.*

Mouth/Throat *Brown bitter coating on tongue. Gums burn.*

Digestion/Appetite Gastric fever.

Cough/Lungs *Pneumonia of left lung and left lower lobe. Pain through lower left lung. Holds chest when coughing.* (Bry.) *Rattling of mucous in chest.* (Ant-t., Ipec., Kali-c.) *Cough with copious thick, ropy greenish expectoration.*

Fever/Chill *Pneumonia of left lung and left lower lobe.* Gastric fever.

Discharges *Thick, green, yellow and copious.*

Position/Motion *Holds chest when coughing.*

Weather/Body Temperature/Reactions *Worse in damp weather and living in damp places. Worse every change to wet weather.* Cannot get warm, chilly and shaking with cold; cold people.

Time/Speed *Worse at 4 am or 5 am.*

NITRIC ACID

Main Indications *Anxiety about diseases.* (Ars-a., Gels.) *Irritable. Fear of death.* (Acon., Ars-a.) *Sticking splinter-like pains. Affects the margin of any outlet such as mouth, eyes and anus. Easy haemorrhages of bright blood, or like bloody water. Smelly.*

Causation Loss of sleep, e.g. from nursing the sick. Spinal injury. Antibiotics, drugs, penicillin and mercury.

Mentals *Anxiety about diseases. Irritable. Fear of death and disease. Can be delirious.*

Appearance/Head/Face/Eyes/Ears/Nose *Head pain like a band.* During headaches *very sensitive to noise. Eyes have sharp sticking pains. Eyes weep.* Photophobia, ulceration of cornea. Face yellow and sickly with peeling lips. *Scabby cracked and raw corners of lips.* Nose bleeding dark and clotted blood *with chest problems.* Chronic nasal catarrh with yellow smelly *corrosive* discharge.

Mouth/Throat *Ulcers in mouth with splinter-like pains. Throat has splinter-like pains.* Bloody saliva, gums spongy.

Digestion/Appetite *Loves indigestible things like chalk and earth.* Worse for milk and fatty food. Averse to meat and sweet things. *Cutting and splinter-like pains after stools.*

Cough/Lungs *Short of breath on going upstairs.* Bloody and/or yellowish expectoration.

Urine *Urine is smelly and strong. Feels cold as it passes.*

Fever/Chill Icy coldness of soles of feet. Chilly continuously. Sweats easily then takes cold.

Pain Type *Splinter-like pains.*

Discharges *Acrid and offensive, thin usually* but can be thick. *Profuse sweats break out on hands and feet. Easy haemorrhages of bright blood, or like bloody water.*

Touch/Pressure *Worse for slight touch.*

Position/Motion *Worse for jarring.*

Light/Dark/Noise *Sensitive to noise.*

Weather/Body Temperature/Reactions *Worse cold air and hot weather.*

Relationship to other remedies Incompatible Lach.

NUX VOMICA

Main Indications Affects liver. *Spasms and over-sensitiveness. Irritability mentally and physically. This remedy is not really indicated for the serious stages of Bird flu but might come in useful for the less serious cases.*

Causation *Bad effects from working late into night, drugs and stimulants.*

Mentals Extremely *cross and impatient, worse when alone. Zealous fiery mood. Can be delirious. Neat and fastidious.*

Appearance/Head/Face/Eyes/Ears/Nose *Nose stuffed up at night and out of doors. Stuffed up feeling and bloody, acrid discharge. Nosebleeds.* Eyes worse for light.

Mouth/Throat *Bloody saliva. Taste bitter. Gums bleed. Throat rough and tickling with stitching pains into ear. Breath smelly.*

Digestion/Appetite *Bruised soreness of abdominal walls, sore bowels, windy and distended. Colic with upward pressure affecting lungs. Frequent and ineffectual urging to pass stool. As if part of stool remained. Passing stool relieves pains for a while but constant unease remains in the rectum. As if a weight in the stomach, food lies heavily in stomach, and pain is worse for eating; windy, belching and tendency to hiccoughs. Pain and bloating several hours after eating. Nausea and vomiting with much retching. Desires fats and stimulants. Better for hot drinks. Gastric fever.* Liver disorders.

Cough/Lungs *Breathing difficulties from pressure from stomach upwards. Shallow and oppressed breathing. Cough brings on headache.* (Bry.)

Extremities/Back *Aching limbs.*

Fever/Chill *Feverish but freezing inside. Must be covered up regardless how hot he becomes. Cannot move or uncover without feeling chilly. Blueness of finger nails. Chill with thirst, heat without thirst. Gastric fever.* Delirium.

Pain Type *Urge to stool with every pain. Spasms. Over-sensitiveness.*

Discharges *Better for free discharges. Acrid, bloody.*

Touch/Pressure *Worse for pressure of clothes.*

Position/Motion *Cannot move without feeling chillier.*
Light/Dark/Noise *Worse for slightest noise, smells and light.*
Weather/Body Temperature/Reactions *Very chilly*, cannot get warm despite heat. (Bell.) *During fever feels freezing inside. Better for hot drinks, worse for uncovering, worse for open air.*
Time/Speed *Worse in early morning, or from 3 am onwards.*
Sleep *Cannot sleep after 3 am. Better for a nap.*

OSCILLOCOCCINUM (otherwise known as Anas.Barb.)
Main Indications Use this remedy *only for simple flu particularly in the early stages,* for which it is an excellent remedy and very useful. While it has been suggested as a possible remedy for Bird flu, it is unlikely to be indicated for the more serious and complicated cases when the patient gets pneumonia and/or if the body starts destroying itself.
Mentals Anxious about dirt and infections, washes hands a lot.
Appearance/Head/Face/Eyes/Ears/Nose Nose running or blocked up. Eyes have *yellow discharge during early stages of flu, conjunctivitis.* Ears inflamed. Head bursting and throbbing, but only during the early stages of flu.
Digestion/Appetite Cramps followed by diarrhœa. Milk and eggs disagree.
Cough/Lungs Loose sounding cough usually.
Discharges *Yellow discharge from eyes.*
Weather/Body Temperature/Reactions Better for warmth.
Time/Speed Only useful in the early stages and for uncomplicated cases.

PHOSPHORUS
Main Indications *Exhausting diarrhœa; lung problems with weight on chest sensation; haemorrhages; nervous exhaustion; always wants company; burning pains. Bleeding from anywhere, urinates blood, nosebleeds etc.*
Causation Exposure to very heavy rain, weather change, going from hot to cold atmosphere or from cold to hot, eating too much salt, putting hands into very cold water, anaesthetic.
Mentals *Excitable and impressionable. Fears to be alone, fears the dark, fears thunder. Loves company, wants to go to the party however ill they are. Sympathetic and loves sympathy. Can be delirious.*
Appearance/Head/Face/Eyes/Ears/Nose *Heat comes up spine to head, coldness of occiput (back of head).* Letters appear red. *Nosebleeds. Photophobia.*
Mouth/Throat *Larynx painful, preventing talking. Voice hoarse. Gums bleed easily.*
Digestion/Appetite Worse too much salt, *desires salt. Desires and is better for cold food and cold drink, but vomits almost immediately as it warms in stomach. Weak, empty gone sensation in abdomen. Diarrhœa with weakness after stool, exhausting diarrhœa. White stool, bleeding with stool.* Gastric fever.

Cough/Lungs *Tight across chest, weight on chest, breathing fast and difficult. Heat in chest. Dryness of air passages. Palpitations with anxiety. Pneumonia with oppression and worse for lying on left side. Affects left and right lung, particularly lower left lobe. Stitching pains in chest on left side, better lying on right side. Whole body trembles with cough. Cough worse for cold air and worse from change of air temperature from warm to cold, or cold to warm. Hard dry cough, racking cough. Thirst for cold water with cough. Rusty or bloody expectoration, tastes salty, sour, sweet or cold.* Hoarse voice worse in evening.

Urine *Sugar in urine, bloody urine.*

Extremities/Back *Joints may give way suddenly, arms and hands go numb, heat between shoulder blades.*

Skin Wounds bleed a lot, even if small.

Fever/Chill Fever and night sweats. Gastric fever. *Septic fever.*

Pain Type *Tightness in chest; weight on chest. Burning pains.*

Discharges *Bloody. Bleeds very easily, bright red blood.*

Side *Worse lying on left side. Affects lower left lobe of lungs mostly.*

Touch/Pressure Desires massage.

Position/Motion *Worse lying on left side*, or on back or painful side, better lying on right side.

Light/Dark/Noise Fear of dark. Photophobia.

Weather/Body Temperature/Reactions *Worse from thunderstorms and lightning; worse warm food and drink; worse from change of weather and change of room temperature. Cold air relieves head and face symptoms, but worsens cough and sore throats. Generally chilly people.*

Time/Speed *Particularly worse at dusk, sudden prostration.*

Sleep Better for short naps. Vivid dreams of fire and blood.

Relationship to other remedies Complementary Ars-a., Nux-v., and Sang. (Incompatible Caust.)

PULSATILLA

Main Indications *(1) Changeable symptoms, both physically and mentally. Pains move around and change from place to place; the type of pains change too. Moods change easily from tears to laughter and back again. (2) Thick bland discharges, usually creamy white, creamy yellow or greenish. (3) Usually warm but chilly when ill, generally worse for warmth and better for fresh air. (4) Thirstless despite having a dry mouth. Digestive upsets. Dependent.*

Causation Suppressions of any discharge or eruption. Being abandoned, grief, eating ice cream, port, fats, pastry and rich puddings. Getting chilled, getting wet feet.

Mentals *Weepy, tearful mood. Worse alone. Affectionate. Mild, gentle, timid people usually. Easily moved to laughter or tears. Changeable mood. Desires a great deal of sympathy and attention. May be manipulative. Fears abandonment.*

Dependent. Can be delirious. Jealousy.

Appearance/Head/Face/Eyes/Ears/Nose *Thick yellow green mucus from nose and ears and eyes. Conjunctivitis. Nosebleeds.*

Mouth/Throat *Tongue covered with yellow or white tenacious mucus. Sweet or bitter taste.*

Digestion/Appetite *Bitter taste and heavy feeling in stomach.* Worse eating rich foods, such as pastry or cream, although these are liked and desired. Dislikes pork. Wants refreshing foods. Worse for greasy foods, worse for warm foods. *Thirstlessness, even with a dry mouth. Windy. Changeable stools. Gastric fever.*

Cough/Lungs *Shortness of breath, worse for warm stuffy room, must sit up to cough, expectoration easy, bland and yellowy green. Pressure and soreness on chest. Cough dry in evening and night, worse on lying down, loose in morning and daytime. Pneumonia.*

Extremities/Back Pains in limbs, pains move around fast and stop suddenly, pains worse for letting affected part hang down.

Fever/Chill *Very much worse for stuffy rooms, desire fresh air. Chill worse around 4 pm. External heat aggravates. With any pains or during any illness can become cold, although they are usually warm and worse in warm air. Gastric fever. Septic fever.*

Pain Type Starts gradually but stops suddenly. Pains wander around from place to place, *constantly changing both place and type.* Relieved by cool.

Discharges *Profuse, bland, thick discharges. Usually yellowish-green or creamy coloured; frequently changeable in appearance.*

Touch/Pressure Better for touch and pressure. Babies and children particularly want cuddles. Usually clingy.

Position/Motion Better moving gently. Better changing position. Worse lying on left side. *Better sitting upright.*

Weather/Body Temperature/Reactions *Usually warm people; they are worse for overheating and can overheat easily. When ill are usually chilly, worse for warm air and desire fresh open air.*

Time/Speed *Worse in the evening/twilight.* (Phos.) *Chill worse around 4 pm.*

PYROGEN

Main Indications *Septic fevers, flu, septicaemia.*

Causation *Blood poisoning. Eating bad meat or fish.*

Mentals *Very restless.*

Appearance/Head/Face/Eyes/Ears/Nose Worse moving eyes. *Nosebleeds.*

Mouth/Throat *Brown streak in centre of tongue, or shiny, dry, large, flabby, fiery red, clean and smooth. Breath smelly.*

Digestion/Appetite *Diarrhœa very smelly, brown or black. Involuntary and painless.*

Cough/Lungs *Neglected pneumonia.* Cough with lots of phlegm, worse in warm room, cough causes burning in larynx and lungs. Cough worse lying, better sitting up. *Heart palpitations; fast pulse, out of proportion to fever, or else very slow. Heart failure in septic states. Can feel and hear pulse in ears, preventing sleep. Pulse quick and out of all proportion to temperature, or the reverse.*

Extremities/Back *Bed feels too hard. Sore limbs.*

Fever/Chill *High fever with sore limbs and delirium Sweat does not cause fall in temperature.* (Merc-s.) *Septic fever.*

Pain Type *Bruised, sore, aching and weak, although restless.*

Discharges *All very smelly.*

Touch/Pressure Better for pressure. Bed feels hard.

Position/Motion Better for walking, motion, stretching and sitting (cough).

Weather/Body Temperature/Reactions Better for heat, better for hot bath, worse for cold, worse for damp.

Relationship to other remedies Complementary: Bry. and Bapt. Compare Rhus Tox., better for stretching limbs.

RHUS TOX.

Main Indications *Affects nerves and spinal cord. Stiffness of muscles and joints. Extremely restless, cannot get comfortable. Flu.* (*Typhoid-like fevers.*)

Causation *Getting cold and wet, damp sheets, getting wet when heated. Strains and over-lifting.*

Mentals *Restless, dreams of great exertion. Fear of poison. Apprehension at night, cannot remain in bed. Can be delirious.*

Appearance/Head/Face/Eyes/Ears/Nose Head *Heavy head.* Pain occiput, brain feels loose and as if striking against skull. Face may be swollen, and jaws crack when chewing. Fever blisters, cold sores. Eyes *Inflammation of eye, swelling of eye and pustular inflammations of eye.* Nose *Nosebleeds.*

Mouth/Throat *Red triangular tip to tongue or diagonally red. Throat feels raw and rough. The voice is hoarse, but improves with talking only getting worse again from over-use. Swallowing solids is difficult.*

Digestion/Appetite *Desires milk, drowsy after food. Very thirsty. Gastric fever.*

Cough/Lungs *Dry teasing cough, worse during chill, worse for putting hand out of bed. Heart palpitations and trembling when still.* Rust coloured sputum.

Extremities/Back *Tearing pains ligaments, muscles and tendons. Stiffness, paralyzed. Back stiff, particularly the small of the back, better for continued motion, better for lying on something hard, may lie on floor. Affects muscles particularly but can have severe aching in bones.* (Eup-perf. but Eup-perf. bone pains are even worse than those of Rhus-t.) *Restless legs and restless trying to find comfortable position.*

Skin Shingles, urticaria, cellulitis, eruptions may be worse under hair.

Fever/Chill *Restless, stiff and sore with fever. Worse for least uncovering. Very chilly, desire to stretch. Pneumonia. Gastric fever. Septic fever.*

Pain Type *Stiff, sore and aching. As if tearing asunder. Cannot get comfortable,* *very restless. Better for hard pressure and massage.*

Side Often worse on left side. May be worse lying on right side.

Touch/Pressure *Better for massage and rubbing. Sleeps on floor as better for hard pressure.*

Position/Motion *Worse for initial motion, better for continued motion, worse over-exertion, worse for rest. Sleeps on floor as prefers lying on something hard.*

Weather/Body Temperature/Reactions *Worse for cold, worse for wet weather, worse slightest exposure to cold and draughts, better for warm bath and better for heat, worse before storms. Worse cooling down suddenly when hot and sweaty.*

Relationship to other remedies (Inimical: Apis.)

SANGUINARIA

Main Indications *Affects particularly the mucus membranes of lungs. Right sided. Burning pains, congestions of blood to head, chest and abdomen, with pulsations. Bilious headaches from missing meals. Pneumonia. Headaches, right sided. Sensitive to, and worse for odours, particularly of flowers.*

Causation *Sudden suppression of catarrh of nose or lungs, may be followed by diarrhœa.*

Mentals Angry, irritable, morose. Stupor, sleepiness, confused. Occasionally optimistic.

Appearance/Head/Face/Eyes/Ears/Nose *Face has red cheeks, often a round circumscribed redness or a hectic flush of cheeks with burning. Head pains that start in morning, increase until noon, then diminish. Bursting as if eyes would be pressed out. Periodical sick headache ascending from occiput (back of head) to over right eye; or like a flash of lightning in occiput, ameliorated by sleep; periodic every 7th day or may be worse during menopause. Rush of blood to head with nausea and faintness. Pain sharp and throbbing, worse for light, vomits at its worst, presses head into pillow. Bilious headaches from missing meals. Sick or faint from smell of flowers.*

Digestion/Appetite Diarrhœa following suppression of catarrh of nose or lungs. *Congestions of blood to abdomen with pulsations. Bilious.*

Cough/Lungs *Cough with gastric problems, better for burping. Burning in chest followed by diarrhœa in pneumonia. Catarrhal pneumonia both sides but worse on right side of lungs. Rust coloured smelly tough sputum, nearly impossible to raise. Spasmodic cough after whooping cough and flu. Difficulty breathing.*

Extremities/Back *Rheumatism right shoulder, worse in night, worse raising arm. Burning palms and soles.*

Skin *Red burning circumscribed blotches* and spots.

Fever/Chill *Pneumonia. Burning pains and congestions of blood to head, chest and abdomen, with pulsation. Worse right side.*

Pain Type *Burning, as if hot water poured over part. Burning in stomach with gastric problems. Burning in chest followed by diarrhœa in pneumonia.*

Discharges Better for passing wind. Better for burping.

Side *Right sided.*

Touch/Pressure Bores head into pillow to try to help the pain, but generally worse for touch particularly right side of body.

Position/Motion Better for lying on left side.

Light/Dark/Noise Worse for light, better for darkness.

Weather/Body Temperature/Reactions Better for cool air.

Time/Speed *Worse at around 3 am.* Worse during night. Worse during menopause. Headaches that start in morning, increase until noon, then diminish.

Relationship to other remedies Complementary to Bell. and Ant-t.

SULPHUR

Main Indications *Itching and redness particularly of orifices; lips, ears, nose, eyelids, anus. Local burning, congestion and throbbing. Flushes of heat. Worse for water although desires it. Relapsing complaints. Septic fevers.*

Causation Suppressions of all kinds. Drinking cold water on hot days.

Mentals *Imagines himself to be a great person. Selfish. Can be delirious. Restlessness.*

Appearance/Head/Face/Eyes/Ears/Nose Hair dry. Nose has dry catarrh, is scabby and easily bleeding. *Very red lips. Eyes bloodshot, red rimmed eyes, conjunctivitis without much discharge but with a lot of watery tears. Eyes are sore, raw, itchy and burning. Restlessness. Face circumscribed redness of cheeks.* (Sang.) Heat, pain and throbbing in top of head.

Mouth/Throat *Bleeding gums, bitter taste in mouth.*

Digestion/Appetite *Milk aggravates. Diarrhœa in early morning drives out of bed. Profuse colourless urination. Gastric fever.*

Cough/Lungs Desires air. *Rattling mucous in chest*, green, sweet, thickish expectoration. Pneumonia in either or both lungs. Loose cough with tickling in larynx. Worse around 11-12 am, usually about an hour before a meal. *Oppression and weight on chest. Burning or coldness in chest.*

Extremities/Back *Hot and sweaty hands and feet.* Soles burn, uncovers them.

Skin *Red orifices anywhere.* Dry. *Itching, worse warmth.*

Fever/Chill *Flushes of heat frequently throughout body.* Dry skin and extreme thirst. Sweat in single parts, or one side of body only. Sweating is worse at night, may smell of sulphur. Sweating without relief. (Merc-s., Pyrog.) Feels too hot. Relapsing fever, septic fever, gastric fever.

Pain Type Itching and burning. Local burning and throbbing and congestion. Rawness.

Discharges Acrid, blood streaked and smelly.

Position/Motion Standing aggravates.

Weather/Body Temperature/Reactions *Worse for warmth of bed, worse for heat generally. Better for dry warm weather. Worse if heated.*

Time/Speed *Worse at around 11 am.*

Relationship to other remedies Helps other remedies to work (if they are well indicated, but despite this symptoms relapse).

VERATRUM ALBUM

Main Indications *Affects nerves. Icy coldness, blueness and weakness. Vomiting and diarrhœa, purging and cramps. Profuse and violent retching and vomiting. Profound prostration. Symptoms violent and sudden. Fainting easily. Copious everything; stools, urine, vomiting, sweat and saliva.*

Causation Post-operative shock, fright, suppressed rashes, grief.

Mentals Indifference, dwells on imaginary impending misfortunes. *Can be delirious.*

Appearance/Head/Face/Eyes/Ears/Nose *Pale, blue and cold. Cold sweat on forehead. As if lump of ice on top of head, icy cold tip of nose and face. Nosebleed from right nostril.*

Digestion/Appetite *Worse for drinking cold water as vomits it at once* (Ars-a., Phos.) *but desires cold water. Strong appetite. Copious vomiting with nausea, worse for drinking and worse for motion.* (Bry.) *Icy cold feeling in stomach and abdomen. Stools large with much straining and copious, violent evacuation. Gastric fever.*

Cough/Lungs Fullness feeling in chest with belching. Mucus in chest with rattling. Chronic bronchitis of the aged. Cough worse entering warm room from cold. (Puls., Phos., Bry.) Cough is better cold drinks. Barking cough with belching. Involuntary urination with cough.

Skin *Cold as death.*

Fever/Chill Rapid changes in temperature with cold or hot sweat. *Gastric fever.*

Pain Type *Cramping.*

Discharges *Profuse.*

Position/Motion *Worse for exertion. Vomiting worse for motion.*

Weather/Body Temperature/Reactions *Extreme coldness and general coldness anywhere. Worse for cold drinks and worse for cold food and cold room; but cough is worse for going into warm room. Cold as death.*

VERATRUM VIRIDE

Main Indications *Violent congestions, particularly of head and face. Pneumonia. Influenza.*

Causation *Sunstroke.*

Mentals *Loquatious, suspicious and/or quarrelsome. Delirium; fury, screams and mutters.*

Appearance/Head/Face/Eyes/Ears/Nose *Face very flushed but pale on sitting up. Pupils dilated. Head Severe pain at back of head and nape of neck area, so can hardly hold head up. Throbbing pains.*

Digestion/Appetite Nausea and vomiting. *Hiccoughs. Spasms.*

Cough/Lungs *Can feel heart beat throughout the whole body. Pneumonia.*

Fever/Chill Rapidly changing from high fever in the evening to chill in the morning. Delirium.

Pain Type Burning. *Throbbing.*

Discharges Cold clammy or hot sweat.

Weather/Body Temperature/Reactions Worse from sun.

Relationship to other remedies Look at Acon. and Gels.

Appendix - Remedy Names

Shortened name	Usual name used	Full remedy name
Acon.	Aconite	Aconite Napellus
Ant-t.	Ant-tart.	Antimonium Tartaricum
Apis	Apis Mel.	Apis Mellifica
Arg-n.	Arg-nit.	Argentum Nitricum
Ars-a.	Ars.Alb. or Arsen.Alb.	Arsenicum Album
Ars-i.	Ars.Iod. or Arsen.Iod.	Arsenicum Iodatum
Bapt.	Baptisia	Baptisia Tinctoria
Bell.	Belladonna	Belladonna
Bry.	Bryonia	Bryonia
Camph.	Camphor	Camphora
Carb-ac.	Carbolic Acid.	Carbolicum Acidum
Carb-v.	Carbo Veg.	Carbo Vegetabilis
Chel.	Chelidonium	Chelidonium
Crot-h.	Crotalus	Crotalus Horridus
Eup-perf.	Eup. Perf.	Eupatorium Perfoliatum
Ferr-p.	Ferrum Phos.	Ferrum Phosphoricum
Gels.	Gelsemium	Gelsemium
Hep-s.	Hepar or Hepar Sulph	Hepar Sulphuris
Ipec.	Ipecac.	Ipecacuanha
Kali-c.	Kali Carb.	Kali Carbonicum
Lach.	Lachesis	Lachesis
Merc-s.	Merc.Sol.	Mercurius Solubilis
Mur-ac.	Muriatic Acid.	Muriaticum Acidum
Nat-s.	Nat. Sulph.	Natrum Sulphuricum
Nit-ac.	Nit-ac.	Nitric Acid
Nux-v.	Nux Vom.	Nux Vomica
Oscill.	Oscillococcinum	Oscillococcinum
Phos.	Phos.	Phosphorus
Puls.	Pulsatilla	Pulsatilla
Pyrog.	Pyrogen	Pyrogen
Rhus-t.	Rhus Tox.	Rhus Toxicodendron
Sang.	Sanguinaria	Sanguinaria
Sulph.	Sulphur	Sulphur
Verat-a.	Veratrum Alb.	Veratrum Album
Verat-v.	Veratrum Vir.	Veratrum Viride

If you feel having so many remedies in stock is too expensive you probably could get away without having Apis, Arg-n., Ars-i., Hep-s., Merc-s., Mur-ac., Nat-s., and Verat-v. in 30s, just have them in 200s.

Printed in the United Kingdom
by Lightning Source UK Ltd.
136349UK00001BA/4-12/P

9 781899 820290